Bruce Fife, N.D.

The Healing Crisis

Third Edition

Piccadilly Books, Ltd.
Colorado Springs, CO

Published by:
Piccadilly Books, Ltd.
P.O. Box 25203
Colorado Springs, CO 80936 USA
www.piccadillybooks.com
info@piccadillybooks.com

Library of Congress Cataloging-in-Publication Data
Fife, Bruce, 1952-
    The healing crisis / Bruce Fife.
    p. cm.
    Includes index.
    ISBN 10: 0-941599-33-7 (pbk.)
    ISBN 13: 978-0-941599-33-7 (pbk.)
    1. Naturopathy. 2. Healing. 3. Nature, Healing power of.
I. Title.
RZ440.F54   1997   97-14626
615.5'35--dc21

Printed in the USA.

All healing comes from within.

CONTENTS ■

CHAPTER 1

WHAT IS A
HEALING CRISIS? ————— ∎

Randy*, 45, had gradually been losing his eyesight as a consequence of diabetes. An operation to improve his sight in one eye had failed, making him near blind in that eye. He refused a follow-up operation in the other eye. He had kidney problems, was constantly fatigued, and for months had been plagued with edema (swelling) in his legs, making walking painful. He had been seeing traditional doctors for several years and had given up hope of regaining his health.

A co-worker suggested he see a naturopath—a health care worker who uses natural methods to stimulate and enhance the body's inherent healing capabilities. Out of desperation he took her advice and made an appointment.

The naturopath told him he could regain a great deal of his health if he put in the effort and agreed to follow a strict diet high in fiber and low in fat, sugar, and chemical additives. Randy was given some herbal supplements and encouraged to begin a light exercise program.

---

*Some of the names used in this book have been changed to protect privacy.

Skeptical that simply changing his diet and activity level would have much of an effect, Randy hesitated to begin the program. He was comfortable in his sedentary lifestyle and convenience-food diet. With encouragement from his wife and co-workers, he started the program on Sunday. He began eating whole, natural foods and, despite the discomfort due to his swollen ankles, he took daily walks in his neighborhood. Wednesday night Randy became violently sick with vomiting and diarrhea. Throughout the night he suffered what he thought was a case of the flu. By the next day symptoms began to lessen. The following day he resumed his normal activities and noticed that walking was easier. To his surprise Randy found that the swelling in his ankles and legs, which had troubled him for many months, was now gone. He also noticed a surge in his energy level, and felt better than he had for a long time. He wasn't totally cured from diabetes or its degenerative symptoms, but he found hope that his health could be improved.

The naturopath had told Randy that he might experience unpleasant symptoms before he actually got better. The so-called "flu" he suffered was actually a reaction resulting from the changes he made in his lifestyle. It is known as the "healing crisis".

When the body experiences dramatic symptoms of cleansing as a result of improved organ function and immune efficiency, it is referred to as a healing crisis—"healing" because it expels toxins and brings about improvement in health, "crisis" because the symptoms associated with toxic removal can be dramatic.

The symptoms of the healing crisis are the same as those of a disease crisis (illness). For this reason, the healing crisis is greatly misunderstood and often believed to be an illness that must be treated to restore health. The healing crisis is a positive event, a sign of improving health. Unfortunately, many people mistakenly view it as a disease crisis. One is the result of the body *overcoming* disease, while the other is the result of the body *succumbing* to disease. There is an important need to make a clear distinction between the symptoms of a disease process and those of the healing process.

The healing crisis is one of the most misunderstood aspects of natural healing. Even many health practitioners, including medical doctors, do not generally understand it. They will treat it as a sickness with medicines that stop symptoms and abort the healing process. Knowing what the healing crisis is, why it happens, when it happens, and what to do about it is of vital importance in reclaiming and achieving better health.

The purpose of this book is to help you understand the healing process and to help you gain the greatest benefit from any natural healing modality you might choose.

Health is a matter of choice, not a mystery of chance.
—Robert A. Mendelssohn, M.D.

CHAPTER 2

NATURAL HEALING ▬

Pain had become a constant companion to 35-year-old Anne Frahm. "It felt as if I were being stabbed repeatedly with a large butcher knife." Pain eventually encompassed her entire back, making it increasingly difficult for her to walk.

Thinking it was the effects of a minor traffic accident, she ignored it for several months, hoping it would go away. When she went to her doctor, he diagnosed it as bursitis—inflammation of tissues around the shoulder joint—complicated by a kidney infection. He gave her medications to treat these conditions, but as the weeks went on her suffering intensified.

Finally, her doctor had her come in for more extensive testing, which included a CAT scan.

"I hate to tell you this," the doctor said after the tests, "but you have advanced breast cancer. You need a mastectomy, and I can fit you in at 5:30 p.m. tomorrow, okay?" The danger was immediate.

Five months before the pain in her back became noticeable, she discovered a small lump in her left breast.

A local health clinic verified the presence of two tiny lumps but told her they were benign, noncancerous.

Within a few months those two little lumps had spread throughout her body. Now tests showed tumors covering her skull, shoulder, ribs, pelvic bone, and along her spine. So aggressively had cancer attacked her body that it had eaten a stress fracture into her backbone.

She had the mastectomy to remove her left breast, along with a tumor beneath it the size of a grapefruit. Chemotherapy and radiation treatments were begun to kill the rest of the cancer. Even with chemo and radiation her chances of survival were slim. Anne and her husband were told that most people who have cancer as advanced as hers die within two years.

After Anne was released from the hospital, she went to the library and researched all she could on the subject of cancer. As she studied, she discovered that people had overcome every form of cancer there was. This gave her hope. "I decided to fight my enemy with every ounce of my being." For the next year and a half, she subjected herself to all that the medical world had to offer in the battle against cancer.

"For a time my cancer count went steadily downward toward remission. Things looked hopeful," Anne said, "but about ten months into treatment, just as my oncologist had predicted, the chemo began to wane in its effectiveness." New drugs were tried. Nothing worked.

As a last resort doctors decided to bombard her cancer with massive doses of chemotherapy, many times stronger than her body could safely tolerate. In attempting to kill the cancer this way, healthy cells, too, are also destroyed. Especially vulnerable are stem cells made in the bone marrow. In order to keep her from dying from the treatment, she would have to have a bone marrow transplant.

Anne would become her own bone marrow donor. Before treatment, stem cells from her blood were saved so that they could be reinjected into her body later to rebuild the destroyed bone marrow.

Anne spent 52 days in treatment. Doctors tested her bone marrow to see if the torture she endured was all worth it.

"I'm so sorry," said the doctor, "there's still a lot of cancer in your bone marrow." Additional chemotherapy would only weaken her more and hasten death. She was told to get her affairs in order; there was nothing else they could do. Medical science had given up on her. She was left to die.

In her previous research on cancer she learned that many survivors had overcome the disease using natural therapies. The standard medical treatments had not worked for her. She decided to take a different approach; she visited a nutritionist who started her on a cleansing diet and detoxification program.

"Five weeks later, tests done by my oncologist revealed no trace of cancer! He was flabbergasted!" Five weeks of cleansing using harmless methods did more for Anne than a year and a half of drugs, surgery, and all of the knowledge of medical science.

The Body's Power to Heal

All natural methods of healing are based on the concept that the body is capable of curing just about any illness if it is given the opportunity—that is, if negative influences such as environmental toxins, emotional stress, malnutrition, etc. are removed.

The body has an amazing capacity to heal itself. When we get a cut, break a bone, tear a muscle, or get a bacterial infection, the body immediately goes to work to repair the damage. We develop symptoms (mucus discharge, fever, coughing, vomiting, diarrhea, fatigue, etc.) to fight and remove harmful substances. The body knows what to do in every case.

Every person that has ever lived and every person that is now living have all been designed from the same master blueprint. There are slight variations in size, shape, color—genetic variation—but the processes by which the body functions, adapts to its environment, and reacts to disease are the same. One process does not operate in one person and a different process in another. There is a master plan upon which all higher forms of animal life operate, and it is universal in nature. This process ensures the survival of the species amongst a sea of disease-causing microorganisms and natural toxins commonly found in the environment.

There have been, and still are, many devastating plagues on the earth that have killed numerous people. But there are people who have survived even the most deadly diseases. "There is no incurable disease from which someone has not recovered," says Bernie Siegal, M.D., author of several books on health and healing, "even at the threshold of death." Our bodies were designed to repair themselves and combat any potentially harmful substance we encounter. If one person has the innate capability to overcome a particular disease, then *all* of us must have that same ability. If healing does not occur, then the body's natural healing processes are blocked—by toxic overload, malnutrition, psychological barriers, excessive stress, etc. Remove these barriers and health will return—it is the law of nature.

The Immune System

The immune system is our body's defense mechanism. It protects us from disease-causing microorganisms, organic and inorganic toxins, and our own cells that are damaged or have turned malignant or cancerous. The immune system is comprised of billions of cells and molecules distributed throughout the body. The backbone of the immune system is the white blood cells and specialized protein molecules such as antibodies and complements.

There are many different types of white blood cells, all of which can be classified under two general categories—lymphocyte and phagocyte. Lymphocytes, at several million strong, are the most numerous cells of the immune system. They continually patrol the bloodstream and interstitial spaces between cells, searching out and destroying foreign molecules. There are two major types: B-lymphocytes and T-lymphocytes, also called B cells and T cells. B cells are the antibody factories of the body. T cells, some of which have the distinction of being labeled "Killer" T cells, defend by tearing or puncturing enemy cells and by injecting a substance that is lethal to the invader but rendered harmless to our bodies. This substance also attracts, in huge numbers, other white blood cells which join in the battle.

The other main type of white blood cell, the phagocyte, attacks and kills invaders by eating them. These jelly-like cells engulf foreign particles, even reaching out with arm-like extensions to grab their victims. Once the invader is consumed, digestive enzymes tear the molecules apart.

How do our white blood cells tell what is foreign and what is not? Each cell in our body displays its genetic code, like an identification badge. White blood cells constantly monitor the genetic badges of every cell they encounter. If the DNA marker on a cell matches its own, it is recognized

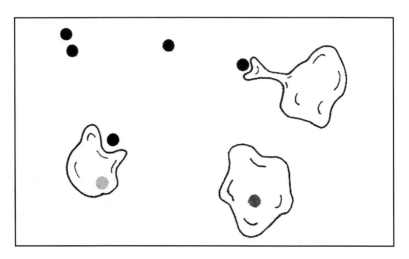

White blood cells (phagocytes) attacking and "eating" bacteria.

as part of itself and left alone. If the DNA doesn't match, it is identified as a potentially dangerous intruder and immediately attacked. In this manner all foreign particles are swept from the body.

Antibodies are one of the most powerful weapons by which the immune system fights invading organisms. When a B cell encounters a foreign substance, it constructs an antibody designed specifically to disable that particular invader. It usually takes a day or two for the B cells to alert others and get antibody production into full swing. During this time invading organisms may multiply in vast numbers, initiating the symptoms associated with illness. If not for the actions of other white blood cells, the body would succumb to this invading army and die within days. When fully activated, B cells can secrete antibodies at the rate of 2,000 per second for several days. These reinforcements join in the battle, putting a relatively quick end to the fight.

Once we have created an antibody to a particular organism, we are said to be immune to it. The B cells keep a memory of the code of these foreign bodies so that if they ever attack again, the right type of antibodies can be quickly reproduced by the millions. This is why people can get measles one time and for the rest of their lives be immune to the disease. Every time someone is exposed to the measles virus, the body bursts into frenzied production of measles antibodies that destroy the invader before disease symptoms can even develop.

Antibodies are uniquely structured to deactivate or kill specific invading cells. An antibody that destroys the mumps virus will not be effective against rhinovirus, which causes the common cold. Although we build an immunity to cold and flu viruses just as we do with the mumps virus, there are numerous cold and flu viruses that are continually mutating and producing different strains. For this reason, we often get several cold and flu infections throughout our lifetime.

Another important type of immune system protein is the complement. Complement molecules are activated by antibody activity. These tiny defending molecules attack invading organisms many times their own size. Complements kill their foe by attaching themselves to the invader's outer membrane layer (the cell wall). Once attached, they drill holes in the invader's membranes, allowing sodium from surrounding fluids to rapidly diffuse into the cell. Sodium draws water in through the holes. The foreign cell swells up with water like an inflated balloon until it explodes. Cellular debris is then gobbled up by phagocytes.

Dead and injured cells are nonfunctional and toxic to our body. They, too, must be removed. Although they are a part of our body, their genetic code—their identification badge—becomes altered, and white blood cells remove them just like any other foreign body. When an injury or localized infection occurs, the body quickly initiates an inflammation response, an important part of the healing process. Inflammation is a process by which blood circulation in a particular area is greatly increased. This allows for the rapid influx of defending white blood cells into the affected area. Damaged cells are removed, along with any infectious organisms that may be present. Healthy cells in the area are stimulated to quickly begin multiplying to replace the damaged cells removed by the white blood cells. In this way injuries or damage by infection are healed.

In like manner, cancerous or degenerative cells are also removed. *All* of us have cancerous cells in our bodies. Although the amount in each of us varies, cancer cells are continually being produced in everyone's body. The reason we all don't develop cancer and die is because the cells of our immune system quickly remove these troublemakers before they become a problem.

The body is constantly patrolled by our white blood cells. They are like a huge biological army that is always on alert, patrolling, checking every cell. Whether the invader is a bacteria, virus, chemical toxin, or degenerative or injured cell from our own body, it is neutralized and removed.

Nature has endowed our immune system with the ability to neutralize or kill and remove almost any type of invading organism. Even the so-called supergerms, potentially deadly strains of bacteria that have become immune to antibiotics, are vulnerable to the defensive actions of the white blood cells. Over time, bacteria can develop a resistance to antibiotics becoming immune to their effects. These antibiotic-resistant supergerms can rapidly multiply, killing their host. Pharmaceutical companies are continually searching for new drugs with which to fight them. Many of the infectious diseases that we thought were under control a couple of decades ago, such as pneumonia and tuberculosis, are surging to deadly proportions because antibiotic treatments are failing against the new supergerms.

Although the supergerms are capable of withstanding antibiotics, they are just as vulnerable to the body's natural defenses as are their weaker cousins. To our immune system there is no difference between normal bacteria and these supergerms.

Potentially deadly organisms that cause bubonic plague, yellow fever, typhoid, etc. can all be overcome by a healthy immune system. This is clearly evidenced by the millions of people who have been infected by these organisms and have survived, with and without the use of medications. The body has the power to overcome all pathogenic organisms. But when the immune system is weakened, even a typical flu virus, which would ordinarily only cause minor symptoms for a couple of days, can become deadly.

When the immune system is overworked or when nutrients essential for the production of healthy white blood cells are lacking in our diets, our immune system cannot adequately do its job, sickness and disease results. If the white blood cells are grossly outnumbered, the disease-causing invaders will overcome. If white blood cells are just barely able to keep daily toxins and pathogenic invaders in check, poisons are easily trapped in tissues and build up over time. These poisons can disrupt normal cellular activity, causing degeneration and further burdening the immune system. Good diet and lifestyle choices are the keys to maintaining a strong immune system. Except for a few extremely rare exceptions, we are all born with the power of achieving and maintaining good health.

Treating Symptoms

In traditional medicine, disease is often viewed as a set of symptoms, and treatment is focused upon removing those symptoms. The problem with this approach is that the symptoms are not the cause of the disease; they are only the body's response to it. Suppressing or masking the symptoms will not cure the disease. Taking a pain pill will not cure a headache, it only deadens the nerves so that the pain is not felt. The cause of the headache remains. Taking cough medicine does not cure chest colds. Sleeping pills will not cure insomnia. Prozac will not cure depression. Ritalin will not cure attention deficit disorder (ADD). Cortisone injections will not cure arthritis. When the cause of the problem is not removed, medication must be used regularly to suppress symptoms.

Removing the symptoms brings about a false sense of well-being and perpetuates the attitude of getting a quick fix to solve medical problems. Drugs provide quick relief to many symptoms of illness but don't do a thing about curing the problem. A lot of drugs are sold and a lot of money is made this way. If people were cured, they wouldn't need the constant supply of drugs, and pharmaceutical companies' profits would fall.

Drugs by their very nature are toxic to the body and add to the toxic body's load, often making health worse. We then can become dependent on drugs to relieve symptoms, while the drugs gradually ensure dependence by weakening the body's ability to heal itself. The *Physician's Desk Reference* lists dozens of side effects to each and every over-the-counter and prescription drug. *All* drugs have adverse side effects! All drugs are toxic to some degree. But people use them because they are perceived as providing the quick fix.

In natural medicine, symptoms are viewed as part of the body's healing process. The body is viewed as being smarter than human intellect; it knows best how to heal itself. Natural healing methods support and encourage the body's own healing forces. This way the symptoms are taken care of as the *cause* of the illness is removed. Because these methods focus on the cause of the problem, their effects on symptoms are not as dramatically noticeable as are drugs. When used properly, natural methods cause no adverse side effects, nor do they load the body with harmful toxins.

Health and Dis-ease

Good health is not simply the absence of disease or pain, but also includes physical, mental, and social well-being. A person can be normal by medical standards but still feel and look unhealthy—an absence of well-being. Many diseases, especially chronic illnesses, do not show up on diagnostic tests until the condition has progressed to an advanced stage. For example, 80 percent of the ability of the pancreas to produce digestive enzymes is lost before clinical symptoms occur and a problem can be detected. The loss in function of the pancreas, however, will adversely affect digestion and nutrient absorption, which in turn will affect the health and well-being of the entire body. So a person can be diagnosed as normal or healthy, yet lack good health because of subclinical conditions. Being healthy includes a feeling of well-being or the absence of "dis-ease". Dis-ease is defined as any form of discomfort caused by cellular or tissue malfunction, sickness, or feelings of ill health that put the body or mind at dis-ease.

Dis-ease can be caused by toxins (biologic organisms, environmental pollutants, metabolic waste, food additives and contaminants, as well as too much dietary fat, sugar, and protein), stress (both physical and emotional trauma), malnutrition (lack of essential nutrients and other elements necessary for optimal health), and poor lifestyle habits (lack of exercise, sunshine, and fresh air). When non-harmful methods are used to correct these dis-ease-causing factors, health is restored.*

We are continually exposed to toxins and other negative factors daily. Harmful chemicals, pollution, and pathogenic microorganisms swarm around us 24 hours a day. Modern society creates undue stress as a consequence of just coping with life. Nutrition depleted fast foods, convenience, and overly-processed foods are the normal fare. We cannot prevent contact with all harmful substances, nor can we stop all toxins from entering our bodies. In fact, it is normal for the body to contain some toxins simply as a by-product of cellular metabolism. But our bodies were designed to neutralize and eliminate these toxic substances as quickly as possible to maintain good health. The immune system, liver, kidneys, and other organs work together to remove harmful substances from the body.

If these were not removed, this waste would poison and kill other cells, leading to massive cellular degeneration, excessive stress on organs and tissues throughout the body, and, eventually, death. The body is fully capable of handling the cleanup and removal of a great deal of toxins with enough reserve strength to fight off infections from

---

*For an in-depth discussion on the genesis of disease and how to overcome it see *The Detox Book: How to Detoxify Your Body to Improve Your Health, Stop Disease, and Reverse Aging* published by Piccadilly Books, Ltd.

microorganisms without serious complications. The food we eat, our stress level, and our lifestyle can either support the body's cleansing process or slow it down. When toxins are being assimilated or created faster than they can be eliminated, the toxic accumulations create an environment in which "dis-ease" develops.

The way to recover health is to rid the body of its toxic overload. Removal of dis-ease-causing agents can lead to a healing crisis. Most any harmless method that strengthens the body's natural healing processes can induce a healing crisis. This could involve switching to better quality foods, taking homeopathic medicines, cleansing the colon, fasting, juicing, or using healing herbs, hyperthermia (heat therapy), massage therapy, acupuncture, reflexology, vitamin therapy, exercise, etc. Most traditional methods of healing that involve the use of drugs, radiation, and surgery do not stimulate a cleansing crisis because, by their very nature, they induce trauma to the body and therefore cause stress and damage. The body's vital energies are channeled toward dealing with this trauma rather than cleansing or healing.

Natural, harmless healing methods, on the other hand, do not cause negative stress but stimulate and enhance the normal function of the body. Heat therapy, for example, increases metabolism so that enzymes, hormones,

---

Definitions

Dis-ease. Any form of discomfort caused by cellular or tissue malfunction, sickness, or feelings of ill health which put the body or mind at dis-ease.

Health. Physical, mental, and social well-being and the absence of dis-ease.

antibodies, and cellular rebuilding are all stimulated into increased action. White blood cells are energized, cleaning out more harmful toxins. Poisons are excreted in perspiration and removed from the body. There is nothing harmful about this process, and healing is accelerated and health improved.

In the process of healing, the body removes toxins— environmental poisons, dead and diseased tissues, pathogenic organisms, and metabolic waste. With the removal of these disease-causing agents and the proper circulation and delivery of healing oxygen and other vital elements, the body manufactures and processes hormones, enzymes, and antibodies, building new healthy tissues as they were designed to do. Health returns.

CHAPTER 3

THE CLEANSING PROCESS ■

The healing crisis is an inherent part of the healing process. Sometimes the crisis is severe as heavy cleansing occurs. At other times the crisis may be all but unnoticeable as cleansing may be operating at a slower pace. But cleansing is occurring—it must occur in order to bring about renewed health.

Every year people come down with colds and flu. We are told that these seasonal illnesses are caused by viruses and are easily spread from person to person. Some people get sick several times a year, while others rarely do so. People can work side-by-side exposed to the same germs, yet some get sick and others don't. Why is this? Why don't all those who are exposed to the cold virus catch colds?

Contrary to popular belief, exposure to germs is not the reason people get colds. Bacteria, viruses, fungi, and other pathogenic organisms are constantly in and on our bodies. They are everywhere, and everybody is exposed to them. For example, the rhinovirus, which causes the common cold, is always present, but we don't all have colds because it is kept under control by our immune system. Rhinovirus can only proliferate and cause problems when the immune system becomes weakened by a toxic overload, by physical or mental stress, or other negative factors. It is a well-established fact that cold temperatures do not cause colds, nor does exposure to other sick people. Colds are passed around only among those people who have weak immune systems. Healthy people with strong immune systems can come in contact with those who have highly contagious diseases without "catching" their illness.

Colds are usually more prominent during the winter because people are less healthy at this time. They eat fewer fruits and vegetables, don't get much exercise, and are cooped up in buildings without healing sunlight and fresh air. Stress also is accentuated in these conditions. When our bodies become overloaded with toxins or burdened with excess stress and our immune system becomes overworked, we become susceptible to the cold virus. When a cold strikes, our bodies attempt to purge the virus and other accumulated filth. Sickness is, in effect, a cleansing process. If the body has the strength and nutrients it needs, then the illness is overcome and the body regains health. Because of the cleansing, we may be healthier immediately after the sickness than before. A condition that causes the body to expel toxins is referred to as a cleansing crisis. Thus, a cold is a cleansing crisis. As you will learn later, cleansing crises can also occur without sickness.

If the body is too weak or adequate nourishment is not provided to fight off the invading germs and cleanse toxic substances, the illness will be prolonged. Nutrients vital to good health may be used up in the process and, if not quickly replenished, the deficiency will lead to some degree of malnutrition and all of its accompanying consequences. The person will still feel sick even after the major symptoms have subsided. These are the type of individuals who are at greatest risk from potentially deadly viruses and bacterial infections.

The symptoms associated with common illnesses are part of the body's natural cleansing process. When our bodies become dangerously overloaded with toxins, our immune systems weaken and we become vulnerable to infectious organisms. When we become sick, our body is telling us to rest so it can focus its healing energies on housecleaning (detoxification). Symptoms of sickness—runny nose, fever, diarrhea, nausea, sneezing, coughing, loss of appetite, etc.—are all processes of cleansing.

When we have a fever, for example, body temperature is elevated as a means of killing invading organisms and sweat out by-products of the cleansing process. Heat also stimulates the production of white blood cells—the powerhouse of our immune system. An increase in mucus production, which causes a runny nose and sinus and throat congestion, is an elimination process. The mucus is carrying away harmful debris cleansed from the body. Coughing is a means by which the body removes garbage from the lungs. Vomiting and diarrhea are processes in which the body cleans out the digestive system. Loss of appetite, aching muscles and joints, and fatigue are symptoms that encourage the body to slow down and rest while the cleansing process is taking place. Rest is necessary as the body needs to focus on purification. Pain tells us that there is a problem in the body that needs attention. A sprained ankle will be painful if used normally. The pain causes enough discomfort that we stop using it or treat it carefully to avoid as much pain as possible. In so doing, the body can properly heal the injury. If pain were not present, even if we knew the ankle was injured, we would probably continue to use it, preventing the ankle from healing properly and possibly causing further damage.

Symptoms we associate with illness are actually beneficial. They are not degenerative but constructive processes. Suppressing symptoms with medications only retards the body's healing processes. For example, when pain is present, there is a problem that needs to be corrected, not ignored or suppressed by drugs. If you took pain relieving drugs for a sprained ankle and then continued to walk on the ankle, you would only be suppressing the symptoms and doing greater harm to the ankle. The pain may, or may not, eventually go away, but the ankle will be weakened and perhaps permanently damaged and cluttered with scar tissue. Because it was not allowed to heal properly, it will be vulnerable to further injury. It may continue to cause irritation throughout life. How many

---

■—— **Definitions** ————————■

Cleansing Crisis. The process whereby the body eliminates disease-causing factors. A general term that can be used to describe either a disease crisis or a healing crisis. Often used interchangeably with healing crisis.

Disease Crisis. The process associated with illness and the body's efforts to remove disease-causing agents and restore health. If the body is weak and unable to overcome illness, death or permanent disability may result.

Healing Crisis. The process associated with heightened cleansing and cellular rebuilding. A sign of improving health. Results in better health as disease-causing factors are removed. Only occurs to the degree at which the body can tolerate without injury and therefore will not cause harm.

people complain of "old" injuries? "My old football injury in my knee was acting up," or "I hurt my back a few years ago, and it aches when I sit for a long time," etc. These are all injuries that were not allowed to heal properly and as a consequence give trouble throughout life. Not only are these tissues or organs weakened physically, but their ability to function and remove metabolic waste and toxins is diminished, thus leading to a build-up of poisons that aggravate surrounding tissue, which may eventually lead to dis-ease.

Just as the suppression of pain will lead to incomplete healing and additional problems in the future, suppression of other symptoms will have a similar effect. When drugs are taken to relieve the symptoms of a cold or the flu, poisonous waste is not eliminated as effectively, the illness lasts longer, and toxins accumulate in the tissue of weak organs or damaged tissues of the body. Toxic accumulations in these organs may lead to more serious disease in the future, resulting in surgical removal of the infected tissue. For example, colds treated with drugs will drive toxins deeper into body where they accumulate. Over time, these toxins build up until the body has another period of cleansing, but this time the cleansing is expressed as influenza because a more severe cleansing must occur. But if drugs are taken to stifle the removal of toxins, they again are driven back into the body and later give rise to a more severe condition like bronchitis. If toxins are still prevented from discharging, then emphysema may develop. In many instances, after suppressing symptoms with drugs for some time, the person's condition worsens to the point where surgery is performed to remove the most offending affected organs. This may save the person from death temporarily, but now the body is permanently crippled, denied a valuable part of the anatomy necessary for optimal health. This unbalance may lead to problems with other organs that now must compensate for the lost organs. Surgical removal of a lung will reduce the amount of oxygen delivered to the blood and the rest of the body. The entire body then becomes oxygen starved. As a result, it cannot clean out toxins as well, and toxins accumulate faster, increasing degeneration of other inherently weak or damaged organs. All of this could be avoided by allowing the body to eliminate toxins naturally.

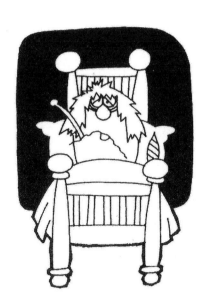

CHAPTER 4

NUTRITIONAL HEALTH ━━━━ ■

"Let thy food be thy medicine and thy medicine be thy food," said Hippocrates (460-377 B.C.), the father of medicine. The old adage "You are what you eat" holds more truth than most people realize. The food we eat supplies the building blocks for our cells and tissues. The quality of the food we consume determines the quality of our health. Long ago in Asia, doctors discovered the connection between health and nutrition. They effectively treated disease simply by adjusting their patients' diets. It is a form of healing that relies on the body's remarkable capacity to repair itself when given the means to do so— that is, when given balanced, natural whole foods free from contamination.

Diet and Health

Diet is the primary means by which health can be improved. According to the World Health Organization, 70 to 80 percent of people in developed nations die from lifestyle- or diet-caused diseases. The majority of cancers are caused by what we put into our bodies. Heart disease, stroke, and atherosclerosis, the biggest killers in industrialized nations, are dietary diseases. Diet is a significant factor in most all degenerative disease. Plainly put, a poor diet leads to ill health.

Many people eat three so-called "balanced" meals a day and falsely believe they should be healthy. Eating too much is a major reason for soaring disease rates in industrialized countries, particularly eating too much refined and hydrogenated vegetable oils, white flour, and sugar. Eating processed convenience foods high in artificial food additives and incidental contaminants also contributes to toxic buildup and stress in our bodies.

Another major cause of dis-ease is malnutrition. Malnutrition is not a just a problem of the impoverished; well-fed people can also be malnourished. Industrialized nations like the United States are full of people who eat plenty but are malnourished because their foods lack the nutrients necessary for optimal health.

Advanced stages of malnutrition can exhibit itself in a number of characteristic diseases such as scurvy, beriberi, marasmus, and others. Such conditions leave the body vulnerable to infections, depress immunity, and stifle healing, normal growth, and body functions. In Third World countries, malnutrition is primarily due to famine, poverty, or politics. In more affluent countries, the problem is masked by the abundance of foods and medicines. In order for symptoms of malnutrition to manifest themselves, a diet must be lacking in essential nutrients for an extended period of time. The body maintains reserves of essential nutrients to protect itself during periods when foods are less readily available. It can take months for signs of malnutrition to become evident. Methods of diagnosing deficiency diseases require malnutrition to be in a relatively advanced stage before it can be detected.

Subclinical malnutrition is a condition where a person consumes just enough essential nutrients to prevent full-blown symptoms of severe malnutrition, but the body is still nutrient deficient and prone to dis-ease. This condition can go on unnoticed indefinitely. In Western countries the problem of subclinical malnutrition is epidemic. Our foods are sadly depleted of nutrients. We eat, and even overeat, but we can still be malnourished because our foods do not contain all the essential nutrients our bodies need to function optimally. As a result, the body can not fight off infections as well, the immune system is chronically depressed, toxins build up, and disease slowly consumes the body. This process is usually attributed to "aging." We are supposed to degenerate and fall apart as we get older and are told there is nothing we can do about it. Often medications are prescribed to mask the symptoms, but taking drugs only adds more chemical toxins to the body.

Subclinical malnutrition is a major problem since it prevents our bodies from removing toxins as it normally should and accelerates the degeneration of the body by toxic buildup. The first thing you should do to improve your health is to provide the body with the nutrients it needs to do the work of internal cleansing and rebuilding.

Definitions

Natural Foods. Whole foods with minimal processing.

Subclinical Malnutrition. A nutritional deficiency in the early stages, before outward signs are apparent.

Building Blocks

The cells in our body are individual living units. Like ourselves, they need nutrients such as water, oxygen, and amino acids to carry on their metabolic processes and fulfill their function. When cells die or become damaged or diseased, they are removed and replaced with new cells. In this way, health is maintained. Cellular replacement is an ongoing process. Some cells last for only a short time while others can exist for years. The cells within the gastrointestinal tract, for example, live only a day or two before they are replaced. Those in the long bones of the arms and legs are completely replaced every seven years or so.

The foods we eat supply our bodies with the nutritional building blocks we need to carry on metabolism and reproduction, as well as making vital substances such as antibodies, complements, hormones, and enzymes, all of which are necessary for life.

Our bodies need some 90 different nutrients in order to maintain optimal health. These nutrients include water, amino acids (from protein), fatty acids (from dietary fats), carbohydrates, vitamins, and minerals. When these nutrients are lacking in our diet, new cells either cannot be made or are constructed with what materials are available, which may make the resulting molecule nonfunctional or even deadly.

Protein synthesis is a good example of the need for all the right materials at the right time. When the body signals a need to build any type of protein (muscle, skin, tendons, blood, hormones, enzymes, etc.), it uses amino acids from the diet. There are 20 amino acids important to human nutrition. At least nine of these are classified as being essential, which means the body cannot manufacture them from other nutrients so we must get them directly from the foods we eat. When the body attempts to build a particular protein, say, for example, an enzyme necessary for digestion of dietary protein, it may need several different essential amino acids to complete the job. If all of these amino acids are available except for just one, the enzyme will not be made. The other amino acids necessary to make the enzyme will be broken down and discarded in the urine. Amino acids are not stored in the body like fat or some vitamins are, so we must have them in our diet continually. Now, since the digestive enzyme is not made, this leads to an enzyme deficiency that hampers the digestive process, limiting the absorption and availability of additional nutrients. A vicious cycle can easily emerge. Without the enzyme necessary to digest protein, essential amino acids that are derived from dietary protein and necessary to build more enzymes cannot be made, and the situation goes from bad to worse.

Our bodies at times will attempt to build certain molecules even when all the right material is not available. Iron is an important constituent in the construction of red blood cells. If your diet is insufficient in iron, and your iron reserves become low, the body will use another element in its place when building new red blood cells. If lead, which is a common contaminant in our environment and our food, is available, our bodies will use it in place of iron in the manufacture of blood. Lead renders the newly formed cells nonfunctional—a potentially fatal situation even in tiny amounts.

A more common problem is the body's use of chemically altered foods in place of natural ones. The use of trans fatty acids provide a good example. Trans fatty acids are dietary fats that have been chemically altered for commercial reasons. They are made by taking unsaturated vegetable oils and saturating them with hydrogen atoms under high heat. This process is called hydrogenation. It is done so the oil can remain solid at room temperature and to extend shelf life. Margarine and shortening are hydrogenated oils. All hydrogenated and partially-hydrogenated oils are damaging to the body.

Hydrogenation changes the shape of unsaturated fatty acid from their natural horseshoe configuration to one that is straight. This is important. Most all of the cell membranes (cell walls), in our body, as well as many other cellular structures, are composed of fatty acids. The cells get the raw materials to construct their membranes from the fatty acids in our diet. If hydrogenated oils are eaten, trans fatty acids from these oils are used as building blocks when cell membranes are made. This is where the shape is important. Normal fatty acids link together in a tight bond because of their horseshoe shape. Trans fatty acids cannot link together or to other fatty acids in the proper manner (see the diagram on the next page). This weakens the cell wall and hampers or even destroys normal cellular function.

If you eat margarine, shortening, hydrogenated and partially hydrogenated oils (found in most processed and convenience foods), or heat-processed refined vegetable oils, then you are consuming trans fatty acids. Every cell in your body may be affected.

Oils are not the only problem. Any chemical food additive has potentially harmful effects. Preservatives are poisons purposely added to foods to kill the cells of microorganisms. If they kill these cells, what are they doing to yours? Their affects on your cells are the same. Artificial dyes, flavor enhancers, anticaking agents, bleaches, and such used in processed foods, as well as pesticides, plastic, and detergent residue and other contaminants all affect the cellular function of our bodies.

If the cells in your body do not function correctly, what happens to you? What happens to your health? Let's look

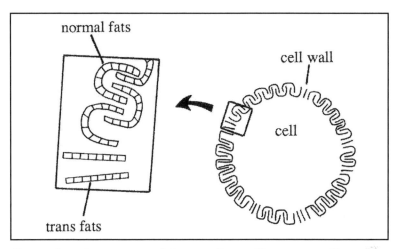

Trans fats incorporated into cells walls causes distortion, adversely affecting cellular function. (Source: Sunlight by Zane R. Kime, M.D.)

at the answer to these questions from the opposite direction. If all the cells in your body were healthy, what would you be? You would be healthy, right? If all your cells were functioning as they should, wouldn't that make the tissues and organs composed of those cells healthy? If all of your organs were functioning with health and vigor, then it stands to reason that you, too, would have good health and vigor.

The opposite is also true. If the cells in your body are weakened by deformed molecules hampering proper function, then the organs composed of such cells will not function optimally and you, as well, will have a lesser degree of health. If your white blood cells, for instance, were composed of faulty materials such as trans fatty acids, do you believe they could effectively fight off infection? Is it any wonder why some people always get seasonal infections while others in the same environment do not?

Or why people develop degenerative diseases, some at young ages, while others remain relatively healthy through old age?

When you give your body clean, healthy foods, you supply it with the building blocks it needs to make healthy cells. Most of us live on diets composed of poor-quality building materials, so many of our cells, and consequently tissues and organs, are inferior to nature's intended design. When you eat good foods, in time, old cells made with inferior materials will be replaced by new healthier cells. There is profound truth in the saying, "You are what you eat." Are you made of the components of wholesome fruits and vegetables, or are you the product of potato chips, soda pop, wieners, and Ding Dongs?

The Key to Effective Healing

Often people will try natural therapies without experiencing any noticeable or long lasting benefit. Such people may even try to discredit these treatments by labeling them as worthless folk remedies based on wives' tales and superstition. The benefit some people get from these treatments, they claim, is a result of the placebo effect and not to any actual healing. This is a common criticism but is totally inaccurate. In most cases, when healing does not occur it is because of neglect to the most important aspect of the natural healing process—the key upon which all natural healing treatments rely in order to be effective.

What is that missing element? Eating a diet composed of nutritious wholesome foods and avoiding dangerous dis-ease-causing additives or contaminants is the key to natural healing. This is why many people who try natural therapies without changing their diets often experience limited results. Take herbal remedies for example. Echinacea is an herb known for its ability to enhance the function of the immune system. A person who eats poorly and takes echinacea to help fight off a cold will only experience limited benefit. As you have seen, trans fatty acids in the diet weaken cell membranes in the body—including the cells of the immune system. White blood cells built with trans fatty acids will be greatly weakened in their ability to fight off the viral infection. Echinacea will not correct this problem. The echinacea may stimulate white blood cell activity, but the white blood cells are not capable of doing their job as nature intended.

Nutrient deficiencies also hamper the body's response to natural treatments. If your diet lacks adequate amounts of vitamin C, you will develop deficiency symptoms that may include anemia, atherosclerosis, depression, frequent infections, bleeding gums, muscle degeneration, joint pain, loosened teeth, and rough skin. Acupuncture, herbs, heat therapy, chiropractic, biofeedback, or most any other natural therapy will be of little help in correcting symptoms associated with a vitamin C deficiency. Vitamin C must come from the diet—a diet rich in fruits and vegetables. A person who eats primarily meats, white bread, and nutrient deficient processed convenience foods is more than likely malnourished or, more correctly, subclinically malnourished. If you lack any of the 90 or so nutrients the body needs, its ability to heal and function optimally is adversely affected.

Chiropractors, acupuncturists, and other natural health care workers often lament over some of their patients who do not get better. Patients may show signs of improvement immediately after treatment, but the improvement is only temporary. Such improvement could be long lasting and even permanent if the person supported it by eating a healthy diet. This is true with any natural treatment. Herbs work better for people who eat healthy foods. Heat therapy, exercise therapy, colon therapy, etc. all work much better when the body is supported with wholesome natural foods and damaging, nutrient deficient foods are avoided.

The most important aspect of any natural healing treatment is diet. Without a proper diet, no other treatment can be completely effective. A good diet just in itself can be a most powerful healer. When combined with other forms of treatment, almost any health problem can be significantly improved, including life-threatening degenerative conditions like cancer, cardiovascular disease, and diabetes.

Natural Foods

Before you start any natural healing program, you must first make sure you are getting the proper nutrition. The most nutritious foods are those which have had the least amount of processing and contamination. These are called natural foods.

From the time food is harvested to the time it ends up on the grocery shelf and in your refrigerator, it can go through many steps of processing. Each step may lower its nutritional value as well as add harmful chemicals.

Food provides the building blocks for cellular regeneration and the syntheses of hormones, antibodies, enzymes, and other essential factors. It is the source for the energy necessary to fuel metabolism and the processes of life. For this reason, it is essential to eat a diet free from chemical additives and rich in nutrients and fiber—as nature intended. The less processing food undergoes and the fresher it is, the more beneficial it is. A natural foods diet is based on whole grains (whole wheat bread, brown rice, oats, etc.) and fresh fruits and vegetables. The food quality chart on pages 42 and 43 lists foods in order of their value to health.

Breaking Addictions

If you have been eating like most people do nowadays, you probably eat a lot of packaged, processed, and convenience foods—all containing numerous food additives. When you switch to more natural foods, you will notice some distinct changes in your health. Be prepared to feel good, bad, and sick. That's right—sick. Before you get better, you may get worse—temporarily.

Ultimately you will be healthier than you have ever been in your life and feel great both physically and mentally. Mental and physical capacity will improve, energy will increase, you will be happier and more positive about yourself and about life. You will lose unwanted fat, improve blood circulation, and look healthier. But before you reach this stage you may experience some physical and psychological changes that may feel unpleasant.

Some food additives, like caffeine and sugar, are physically and psychologically addictive. After eating them for a time, our minds and bodies begin to crave them. It's similar to drug or alcohol addiction. Cravings are one sign of addiction. If we just *have* to have a Pepsi or a candy bar, it is not the body saying it needs the nutrients in these substances; it's the addictions we have to them that initiate this response. Suddenly cutting them out of your diet can cause withdrawal symptoms such as headaches and mild depression or anxiety, which may last a few days. Withdrawal symptoms are a result of the cleansing action of the body—the healing crisis.

Meats as well as food additives stimulate the body and the senses. Meat has a stimulating effect that forces the heart to beat faster than normal, producing a sense of exhilaration. When these foods are reduced or eliminated from the diet, the heart and body slow down to a normal pace, which registers in the mind as relaxation or a decrease

■ Food Quality Chart ■

Level One

Unpolluted spring or filtered water stored in glass container

Fresh organically grown fruits and vegetables

Organically grown whole grains (wheat, rice, oats, corn, spelt, rye, buckwheat, quinoa, amaranth, barley, millet, etc.)

Bread and flour products made from organic whole grains without sugar, preservatives, or chemical additives

Organically grown legumes (dried beans, lentils, split peas, etc. but *not* soy)

Hot whole grain cereals (oatmeal, cracked wheat, bear mush, etc.)

Raw, organic goat milk and cheese

Raw, organic cow milk and dairy products

Game meats (deer, elk, buffalo, pheasant, etc.)

High mountain or deep sea fish (trout, cod, flounder, halibut, etc.)

Organically raised beef, lamb, chicken, and turkey

Organic, free-range eggs

Coconut oil, olive oil, and organic butter

Nuts and seeds (almonds, coconut, sesame seeds, pumpkin seeds, etc.)

Organically grown herbs and herbal teas

Fresh or dried herbs, spices, and herbal seasonings

Organic soured milk products (yogurt, cottage cheese, buttermilk, kefir)

Sea salt or unrefined salt (no additives)

Dried organically grown fruits without preservatives

Bottled organic vegetable and fruit sauces (tomato sauce, spaghetti sauce, apple sauce, etc.)

Organically grown fruit and vegetable juices stored in glass containers (no additives)

Non-organic produce (thoroughly washed or peeled)

Level Two

Frozen vegetables and fruits

Bottled water stored in plastic containers

Natural milk substitutes (soy milk, rice milk, and nut milk)

Natural sweeteners (molasses, raw honey, unprocessed maple syrup, brown rice syrup, and sucanat)

Soybeans and soy products

Cold processed vegetable oils

Condiments made with natural products and without chemical additives

(mayonnaise, salad dressings, tamari sauce, apple cider vinegar, etc.)
Health food store packaged foods without preservatives, chemical
   additives, or hydrogenated oils

Level Three ───────────────────────────────

Canned fruits and vegetables
Conventionally raised meat, fowl, dairy, eggs, shellfish, and bay water
   fish
Pasteurized, homogenized milk and dairy
Refined flours and bread products
White rice
Salt, artificial flavor enhancers, and condiments (soy sauce, mustard,
   catsup, mayonnaise, white wine vinegar, packaged gravy, taco
   seasoning, etc.)
Refined sugar (white sugar, brown sugar, corn syrup, dextrose, sucrose,
   fructose, processed honey, etc.)
Processed vegetable oils (canola, corn, soybean, etc.)
Convenience foods and foods with artificial or chemical additives and
   refined sugars (frozen pizza, TV dinners, pot pies, macaroni and
   cheese, chili beans, beef stew, soup, chips, etc.)
Foods with high refined sugar and/or fat content (candy, sugary
   breakfast cereals, cake, pie, donuts, ice cream, etc.)
Lunch meats (pepperoni, ham, bologna, hot dogs, etc.)
Beverages with high sugar or caffeine content (soda pop, cocoa, coffee,
   black tea, etc.)
Restaurant foods (especially fast food)
Alcohol (hard liquor, wine, beer)
Artificial sugar substitutes (Nutrasweet, Splenda, saccharin, etc.)
Hydrogenated and artificial oils (margarine, shortening, olestra, etc.)

■───────────────────────────────

The foods listed on this chart range from the highest quality at the top
down to the lowest at the bottom. Quality is defined here as the amount
of nutrients contained, amount of processing involved, and amount of
additives or contaminants included.
• Foods in Level 1 should comprise 90 to 100 percent of your diet.
• Foods in Level 2 should comprise no more than 10 percent of your
   diet.
• Foods in Level 3 should comprise no more than 5 percent of your
   diet. You would be best off not eating any of the foods on this level.
   But if you do, keep it to special occasions—definitely not every day.

in energy. This initial letdown, or feeling of lack of energy, will last from one to two weeks. After the body has had time to adjust, you will have a feeling of increased strength and greater well-being as a result of the recuperation and cleansing that follows.

Processed foods with additives and flavor enhancers tend to be more stimulating then natural foods. The first negative feeling you will experience when you switch to a more natural diet is cravings for the highly flavored foods to which you have grown accustomed. Our sense of taste has been overly stimulated as a result of eating too much salt, sugar, flavor enhancers, artificial flavorings, etc. Eating the comparatively bland diet of fresh fruits and vegetables, without additives, can seem dull, and at first perhaps even monotonous (although there are numerous ways to prepare a variety of delicious tasting natural meals). As you become accustomed to eating naturally, your sense of taste will improve, and you will no longer need as much salt to enhance flavor. Rich foods you may have craved before will no longer hold power over you.

The food cravings, possible headaches, temporary drop in energy level, and the perceived blandness from the lack of stimulation from food additives are difficult for some people to handle. Eliminating favorite junk foods is probably the most difficult challenge. It is important to keep a positive mental attitude. If you eat a healthy diet begrudgingly and torture yourself with dreams of cakes, ice cream, and white bread, you will only make yourself miserable! Tell yourself that you don't miss those unhealthy foods and you don't want them. Look for ways to prepare what you can eat so that it satisfies your taste. Eventually, you will begin to enjoy and even prefer natural foods.

"It Didn't Work for Me"

Some people will half-heartedly try to improve their diet for a few days or even a week and then quit. After trying a cleansing diet for several days, John experienced a loss of energy, food cravings, headache, and a general "blah" feeling. He was convinced that a reduction of meat in his daily diet was one of the problems. He worked hard and needed his protein. Eating whole grains, fruits, and vegetables was overrated, he reasoned. It didn't help him; in fact, it made him feel worse.

Cravings for the foods John used to eat were tempting, and when co-workers invited him to join them for lunch, he couldn't resist. For the first time in more than a week John ate junk food—hamburgers, fries, and a Coke. That afternoon his headache went away, he had a boost of energy, and felt better than he had for days. The diet hadn't helped him, he thought, it only made him feel sick. He felt much better eating the way he used to. He was convinced this "health food" diet was just a bunch of baloney. That evening he announced to his wife that he wasn't going to eat rabbit food any more because it made him sick, and besides, he enjoyed eating lots of meat and sugary foods.

Many people experience the same feelings—once they begin to do something healthy, they feel miserable. Even doctors and other traditional medical professionals don't understand this and often point a criticizing finger at some natural product or food and declare it unhealthy because it causes bad reactions. Frequently, they blame the unpleasant reactions to an "allergic response" or "food intolerance" because they have no other explanation.

What really happens is that the body, once it is supplied with vital nutrients and cleansing elements, begins to clean house. Improved health allows the body to remove toxins that bring on symptoms of cleansing. These symptoms can be uncomfortable while they last. When John ate his cholesterol-filled hamburger, grease-dripping fries, and sugary chemical-laden Coke, his body stopped cleaning out the toxins from previous burgers and fries and focused on the more immediate danger. The cleansing symptoms stopped as the body diverted its energies to dealing with his toxic lunch. This gave John a false sense of well-being. The cleansing reaction is a healing process, and healing can't take place while the body is trying to survive.

John is a prime candidate for heart disease, stroke, cancer, or any number of diet-related degenerative diseases.

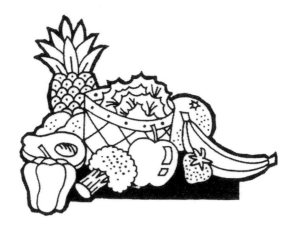

CHAPTER 5

HOW THE HEALING CRISIS WORKS ▪

Curtis was in near shock. The lab tests verified his doctor's suspicion—colon cancer. Curtis had been experiencing abdominal pain and constipation for some time. He knew something was wrong, but he didn't think it would be cancer. No one else in his family ever had cancer.

His doctor recommended surgery to remove the cancerous tumor that was growing on his colon, encouraging him to have it done before it progressed any further. The doctor was persistent, "It's not going to get any better, the sooner we operate the sooner you can recover."

"Will surgery remove all the cancer?" Curtis asked.

"We can remove the tumor," the doctor said, "but there is no guarantee that the cancer hasn't spread to other parts of your body. The concern right now is removing that growth."

"You mean, Doctor, that even if the tumor is removed, I may develop cancer again?"

"Yes, but we will put you on a program of radiation and chemotherapy to inhibit additional growth."

Curtis wanted time to think about it. The prospect of having surgery as well as radiation and chemotherapy did not set well with him.

"Don't wait too long," the doctor warned, "it will only get worse."

With encouragement from a friend, Curtis sought a second opinion from a doctor who believed in and practiced natural therapies. Curtis indeed did have cancer, but this doctor told him he could get rid of it without surgery, without radiation, and without chemotherapy. Cancer throughout his entire body could be expelled so that he wouldn't need to worry about a recurrence. All he had to do was to watch what he ate and follow a special diet program, a diet that consisted of whole, natural foods. Eating "health" foods was a much more pleasant prospect than the dangerous and expensive treatments the first doctor had recommended.

The first things Curtis cut from his regular diet were meat, dairy, and products made with refined sugar and white flour. His new diet consisted primarily of whole grain breads and cereals, fruits, and vegetables. All processed and packaged foods containing food colorings, preservatives, and other chemical additives were out.

He had been warned that removing these poor quality foods from his daily diet and replacing them with nutritious natural foods would have a dramatic affect on his health and well-being. He should not expect immediate recovery. The body needs time to heal. As it cleans and pulls out toxins, he was told, he may experience some discomfort, symptoms similar to sickness. This would not be an adverse reaction caused by eating the healthy foods he was now consuming, but a result of the body purging toxins from the tissues and cells of his body. It would be in fact, a sign that he was getting better, not worse. With that warning, Curtis plunged into his detoxification program.

During the ensuing months, Curtis continued to experience pain and constipation caused by the tumor. Two months after starting his new diet he became ill. He had a fever, was vomiting and was experiencing abdominal cramping and diarrhea. At first, he assumed he had caught the flu. He became worried when he saw blood in his stool. He called the doctor, thinking perhaps the cancer was getting out of hand. His doctor reassured Curtis that as long as he was following his dietary recommendations, he was okay. The "flu" he was experiencing was actually a "healing crisis" in which the body purges poisons from the system. During this time stored toxins can be expelled through any and every orifice in the body. Thus, the vomiting and diarrhea were part of the cleansing process and nothing to be worried about. In fact, it was a good sign because it indicated that the body was getting stronger and healthier. Toxins that had been accumulating in his body for years as the result of a weakened immune system were now being pulled out of the tissues and expelled.

Sure enough, the symptoms he experienced subsided and left after a couple of days. Then the strangest thing happened. Once the symptoms passed, he felt better than he had in years. He seemed to have more energy and a renewed sense of well-being. But his ordeal was not over. The tumor was still there.

Three months later he came down with a severe "cold" with its accompanying sinus congestion, cough, fatigue, headache, and nausea. He had heavy mucus discharge from his lungs and sinuses. Again, the doctor told him not to worry, for it was just another healing crisis. When these symptoms cleared, Curtis noticed an interesting development in his health. Hay fever, which had always bothered him during the summer months, was no longer present. He felt better than he had for a long time. Maybe, he thought, the diet was doing him some good. The tumor, although still present, at least had not gotten any bigger.

In the following months, Curtis experienced several minor healing crises, including a skin rash that broke out over much of his body and lasted several weeks. During this time, his doctor had him go on periodic juice and cleansing fasts and take herbal supplements to accelerate detoxification and healing. Most of his juice fasts lasted from three to seven days. His last fast extended to 36 days and was accompanied by daily enemas.

One morning he woke up with severe diarrhea and agonizing abdominal cramping. His head was pounding and body burned with a fever. During that day he passed, through his bowels, a fleshy tumorous growth the size of his fist covered with long stringy tentacles. This was the tumor that had caused him so much trouble, the tumor the first doctor wanted to remove by surgery. His body removed the tumor on its own, as verified by subsequent examination.

Curtis was freed from the cancer that attacked his body and threatened his health. Not only was the cancer gone, but so was his hay fever, persistent psoriasis that had plagued him for the past several years, and chronic lower-back pain. His bowel movements also became regular and easy. His blood pressure, at one time high, was now normal. He also said his eyesight had improved. He had much more energy and didn't tire as easily as he had just a year before. His whole body, it seemed, was rejuvenated. He felt like he was 20 years younger.

The interesting part about Curtis' story is that his body was able to heal and repair itself—it didn't take medications or surgery. His body did it on its own when harmful substances were removed from his diet and when he was supplied with nutritious foods. If his body knew how to heal itself from cancer and other degenerative conditions, then your body has the same ability. Our bodies are all designed alike. If someone else has been able to overcome a debilitating illness, so can you. Stories like Curtis' are not rare. People are ridding themselves of disease all the time in similar fashion.

All those who have lived on processed and packaged foods, meat, and dairy products sold at grocery stores and in restaurants will go through what is called a healing crisis when they begin to eat healthfully. The healing crisis can also be initiated by any number of natural healing modalities. The healing crisis is the most pronounced part of the cleansing process. You may feel great for a while and then become sick—headaches, stomach cramps, skin eruptions, and aches and pains throughout the body. This healing crisis may occur within a couple of weeks after you start a cleansing program or may not show up for several months. The crisis may repeat itself several times followed by periods of increasingly better health.

This is an area of confusion for many people. After eating healthfully they would expect to get better, not sick. The diet is supposed to make them healthy; why then, are they getting sick? These symptoms of illness are actually indications of improving health.

Toxic Accumulation

One of the major threats to health is toxic accumulation. We are exposed to toxins in the air we breathe, the water we drink, the food we eat, and even in things we come in contact with. As a by-product of metabolism, our own bodies produce toxic substances. If allowed to stay in the body, these toxins would poison the body, and we would become sick and eventually die. That is what is happening to many of us. Environmental toxins (pesticides, industrial chemicals, etc.), biological toxins (microorganisms, parasites, etc.), metabolic toxins (carbon dioxide), dietary toxins (preservatives, artificial colorings, etc.) are continually bombarding and attacking our body. Our immune system feverishly works to expel these potentially deadly toxins. But the more we are exposed, the greater the buildup in our bodies, the more our immune system becomes overworked and less efficient. Dis-ease develops.

Body fat is a primary site for toxic accumulation. When the body forms fat cells, the chemistry of the fat reflects the internal environment of the body at the time of formation. If you are taking medications, traces of those drugs will be incorporated into the fat tissue. If you have a viral or bacterial infection, these may also be trapped in or around the developing fat cells as well as other body tissues. Here these toxic agents may lie dormant until the fat is absorbed. Researchers have identified drugs that have been trapped in body tissues for decades.

Dr. Douglas Lewis, N.D.* described a classic example of old drug residue being released during natural therapy. One of his patients was being treated at the Natural Health Clinic using hyperthermia (sweat therapy) produced with a steam cabinet. The patient had a long history of oral and intravenous drug abuse. After a short period of heating, the

---

*The letters "N.D." following a person's name indicates one who is trained as naturopathic doctor. Unlike medical doctors, naturopaths do not use drugs or surgery but rely on natural healing methods such as nutrition, herbs, exercise, bodywork, etc.

old drug accumulation was released, and he became "high" as a result of the drugs rushing through his bloodstream. Several times during his first few treatments he became incoherent and babbled away about nothing in particular. Gradually over several sessions, this reaction diminished to almost nothing.

Drugs and environmental toxins, including pesticides and food additives, are often stored in the adipose (fat) cells of the body. Storage of these toxins is cumulative, beginning with the smallest intake. These harmful chemicals become lodged in all the fatty tissues of the body. When the body draws upon these reserves of fat for energy, the poison is released into the bloodstream. A New Zealand medical journal provided the following example.

A man undergoing treatment for obesity, which included a sharp reduction of calories in his diet, suddenly developed symptoms of poisoning. On examination, his fat was found to contain substantial amounts of stored dieldrin (a pesticide), which had been metabolized as he lost weight. Over the years, his body had accumulated the toxin from his food and environment.

Some people may reason that if stored toxins are released as a result of dietary changes, maybe it isn't safe to lose excess weight. Losing weight may, in fact, be a health hazard. It might be safer to let these toxins remain locked up in the adipose tissue where they will not do any harm. These people can then continue with their life-destroying habits secure in the belief that drugs and environmental poisons are doing them no great harm.

The adipose tissue, however, is not merely a place for the deposition of fat (which makes up about 18 per cent of the weight of a normal sized person) but has many important functions with which the stored poisons may interfere. Also, fats are widely distributed throughout the organs and tissues of the whole body, even being primary constituents of cell membranes. Therefore, fat-soluble toxins, such as many insecticides in common use, become stored in individual cells, where they are in position to interfere with the most vital and necessary functions of oxidation and energy production. If our cells cannot function properly, then hormone and enzyme production will be adversely affected, as will tissue repair and regeneration. Cells become oxygen deficient, which leads to degeneration and disease. Adipose tissue isn't the only area where microbes and chemical residue can collect. Nerve and other cells may also harbor these dis-ease causing agents.

The Purging Process

During the cleansing process, excess fat, hardened mucus, and toxic wastes throughout the body emulsify and wash out into the bloodstream to be discarded. This influx of toxins into the system brings on symptoms of sickness. People who have had problems with skin rashes or eruptions will frequently eliminate poisons through the skin and new rashes will develop. The skin, as a cleansing organ, is becoming more active. Since the body does not have to spend energy on hard-to-digest junk food, it's able to remove poisons more rapidly. The symptoms will vary according to the materials being discarded, the condition of the organs involved in the elimination, and the amount of energy you have available. You may experience some constipation, occasional diarrhea, frequent urination, nervousness, irritability, depression, fever, mucus discharge, cramps, cold sores, headaches, body aches, boils, skin rashes, infections, swelling, nausea, canker sores, fever blisters, excess gas, tiredness, etc. You will experience discharges from every orifice as the body purges impurities from the system. This is nature's way of cleansing the body.

Surgeons performed a quadruple bypass on Peggy Good, 68, to rescue an ailing heart. Two years later, they went in again; this time to remove a grapefruit-sized tumor—a product of ovarian cancer. They removed some of the tumor, but left some behind. Too risky, they said. Too close to vital organs. Chemotherapy was the next step.

That wasn't the end of it. She developed diabetes. Discouraged, the doctors said she had two months to a year to live. After five sessions of chemotherapy, Peggy, couldn't stand the misery of the therapy any longer and told doctors she preferred to die in peace.

"I was not even human," she says. "I was sick to my stomach, I had headaches, fevers, I was not eating. I was going downhill very fast in the five months I was taking chemo."

She heard about an herbal tea formulation called Essiac that apparently worked magic on terminal cancer victims. She was curious. She reasoned that she had nothing to lose and everything to gain. She began drinking it.

After six weeks of treatment, a frightening event took place in the middle of the night. "I'm wetting the bed," she thought. She looked under the covers. Thick, grayish matter poured from her vagina. "It looked like scum, like pus," she said. Over the next couple of weeks her bowels excreted "awful stuff," sometimes two feet long and an inch and a half in diameter. A feeling of health and well-being enveloped her. "It's hard to explain to people. It's too unreal," she says. "I started to feel so good. I felt better than I had in the last 10 to 15 years."

When she returned to the cancer clinic for an examination, the doctor was shocked. According to him, just a few months ago she was on her death bed with no hope of recovery. Now, stunned, he quietly said, "I'm giving you a clean bill of health," and walked out. "He didn't ask me what I had taken or what I had done. I was left muttering to myself. I would gladly have told anybody if they'd asked, but nobody seemed to care."

In the days that followed, she started having a reaction to the insulin injections and slowly went off the needle. "All I know is that I take nothing for diabetes now." After cleansing dis-ease-causing substances from her body, she regained life and health.

Bob, a successful businessman, had suffered for more than 20 years with pain. Doctors had diagnosed stones in his gallbladder, which was confirmed by x-rays taken with and without idophthalein, a dye used to detect this problem. He hadn't done much to rectify the problem because of his fear and aversion to having an operation, so he quietly suffered year after year.

When Bob heard that juice therapy had been successful in helping others with gallbladder troubles, he jumped at the chance to treat his problem without resorting to surgery. He entered a clinic run by Dr. Norman W. Walker, a juice and natural health advocate. Here he was told that fresh fruit and vegetable juices had powerful cleansing and healing properties that might cause more agonizing pains than any he had suffered before. Dr. Walker explained to him that they would be of brief duration—a few minutes or, perhaps, an hour or so at a time, and would eventually cease altogether with the passing of the dissolved calcium.

Bob drank ten or twelve glasses of hot water with the juice of one lemon in each throughout the day and about three pints of carrot, beet, and cucumber juice daily. "On the second day," Dr. Walker describes, "he did have some terrific spasms of pain for 10 to 15 minutes each. By the end of the week the crisis arrived and for about half an hour he rolled on the floor in agony; but the pain suddenly left him and a short while afterward stones passed out and caused a reaction like mud in his urine. That evening he was a different man. The next day he took a long trip— from New York to Washington and on to Canada—with me in my car, feeling 20 years younger and marveling at the simplicity of nature's miracles."

A Continual Process

Crises are usually short bursts of intense biological activity that propel you to a new level of improved health. A single healing crisis will not purge from your body all the toxins that have accumulated over the years. Many levels must be scaled before optimal health is obtained, but each new level is better than the last and a step closer to total well-being and vitality.

The healing process works in cycles. You will have feelings of health and well-being separated by periods of discomfort caused by the elimination of toxins. If you have had problems with psoriasis, when you improve your diet and start a cleansing program, it may greatly improve the condition, although not completely clear it up. You may be relatively free of skin problems for a couple of months and feel the new way of eating is slowly working. Then, red, itching, flaking skin will suddenly reappear and become as bad, if not worse, than it has ever been before, even though your diet is clean. Your first thought is that you are having a resurgence of the skin problems you've had for years. It may last a month or more but then clear up completely. After this, you will feel and look great. The dry, flaky skin rash was the body's way of ridding itself of toxic debris. Now that the diet is clean, new toxins are not being infused into the cells and tissues, and the body is finally able to purge them from the system.

A few weeks later you may develop a severe case of acne that gets worse over a matter of days, but subsides and clears up in a couple of weeks. Immediately after this, you find that you are free of hepatitis, and you feel more energetic than you were before. The acne served as an outlet for the poisons in the liver which produced the hepatitis.

You will continue to feel good for a time then suddenly become tired and nauseous for a few days. When discomforting symptoms leave, you will feel better than you did before. Still later, you may have a headache, diarrhea, or a fever, but in a day or two you will feel even better than before.

Some healing crises are rather mild and may go almost unnoticed. Others may be quite severe and require bed rest for several days. This is how recovery works. Although you may encounter several minor crises, the first major cleansing crisis is often the worst, with each succeeding reaction being milder and of shorter duration than the one before. The body becomes purer, stronger, and healthier with longer periods of symptom-free health, until you reach a plateau where you are relatively free of symptoms and illness.

CHAPTER 6

HERING'S LAW OF CURE ∎

While your body is cleansing, you will reexperience many of the illnesses you have had in the past, all the way back to childhood. This is called the "reversal process." In the 19th century a Hungarian homeopathic physician named Constantine Hering made a discovery that is now known as Hering's Law of Cure. He stated, "All cure comes from within out, from the head down, and in reverse order as the symptoms have appeared in the body." In other words, healing starts from the inside of the body and works outward, and from the top of the head and works downward, occurring in the reverse order in which sickness afflicted the body. This law has proven accurate since it was first revealed more than a century ago.

From Within Out

Current medical philosophy assumes that if symptoms are absent, the body is healthy and well. Consequently,

*Healing
progresses from
the deepest part
of the body to the
extremities,*

treatment is focused on eliminating symptoms while
ignoring the underlying cause. Symptoms, however, are
reactions of the body in an effort to fight off illness
or disease within the body; they are not illnesses in
themselves. A fever is a symptom, not a disease. Likewise,
a runny nose, diarrhea, high blood pressure, skin rashes,
menstrual disorders, stiffness in the joints, etc. are all
outward signs of disorder inside the body. Treating the
symptom will not cure the disease; drugs may mask the
symptoms, but the underlying cause goes unchecked and
will continue to cause greater problems and resurface later.
Arthritis, for example, is not a localized problem, but a
metabolic or chemical dysfunction of the entire body. In
order to get lasting relief from arthritis, the entire body
must be put back into chemical balance. Drugs that treat
only the area of the joints provide only temporary relief
without curing the problem. Treating localized areas with
drugs, surgery, or radiation is only treating the symptom
and will not bring lasting relief.

Hering's Law states that all cure "comes from within out," which means that in order to get rid of symptoms, you must get rid of the underlying cause. When the body is being healed from the inside, the outward signs (e.g., the symptoms) will disappear. A cleansing diet will strengthen the body so that it can heal itself from the inside out.

From the Head Down

Tanya suffered from multiple sclerosis (MS), a disease in which the coverings on nerves degenerate, impairing nerve function and muscle control. There is no cure for it. After years of unsuccessful treatment from doctors, Tanya was told to accept her fate and live with it. In desperation, she turned to alternative health care.

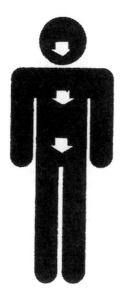

Healing progresses from the upper part of the body to the lower parts of the body affecting emotional and mental aspects first, then the physical.

First, she cleaned up her diet and discontinued all medications. Then she started a series of detoxification programs to cleanse her body of poisonous accumulations of drugs and environmental chemicals.

While she was following the regimen given her, she became angry, bitter, and stressed for no apparent reason. She snapped at her husband and family and didn't know why since they had done nothing particularly wrong.

The most surprising part about the cleansing crisis is that in addition to the physical crisis, there is also an emotional crisis. Just as old illnesses return, emotional disturbances will also resurface. Your past feelings, emotions, thoughts, and memories, will be brought to the foreground. "All cure comes . . . from the head down," as stated by Hering.

Our minds are affected by all the foods, drinks, drugs, and other substances we come into contact with. Schizophrenic and other abnormal behavior including depression, irritability, anger, anxiety, fear, etc. can be caused by nutrient deficiencies and toxicities. The obvious example is what hallucinogenic drugs can do to the mind. The lack of vitamin B_3 can cause schizophrenia-like reactions. Brain allergies cause mental dysfunction (perceptional distortions, thought changes, lost of reason, lapse of memory, irritability, etc.). Often, certain foods will involve brain allergies that manifest themselves in abnormal behavior.* Milk is one of the most common allergens.

Abram Hoffer, M.D., Ph.D., describes the connection between diet and mental health in the book *Medical*

---

*The effects of food on mental and emotional health is well documented in *Brain Allergies* by William H. Philpott, M.D. and Dwight K. Kalita, Ph.D.

Applications of Clinical Nutrition   In one case, a man diagnosed with severe thought disorder, anxiety, and depression had been in and out of mental hospitals for 20 years. He came to Dr. Hoffer for treatment. Dr. Hoffer suspected a dietary problem and put him on a four-day water fast. "On the fifth day," Dr. Hoffer relates, "to my surprise, he was normal; he was free of hallucinations, was no longer paranoid, was not depressed or tense. I then began to test foods, giving him first a glass of milk. Within one hour he was sick mentally and physically, all his psychotic symptoms reappeared and he also suffered nausea, abdominal cramps, and diarrhea. The next day he was better. I told him he was allergic to milk and would have to eliminate all milk products."

When the body begins to cleanse, toxins that have been stored in tissues are released and circulate throughout the body. These substances could involve allergic reactions both physical and mental. Food allergens, medications, and recreational drugs may be released into the bloodstream as the body purges toxins from its tissues. Dr. Hoffer's patient described above was allergic to some chemical element in milk. If that element were stored in his body, upon release due to cleansing, he would experience mental disturbance even though he had not consumed any dairy.

R. H. Van Wyck, director of the Vancouver Institute of Applied Psychology says, "Each physical state is accompanied by a psychological counterpart, and strictly psychotrauma or heavy emotional material is also reexperienced during the reversal and healing crisis process." He has observed that a patient's ability to improve behaviorally is linked to the level of toxic accumulation. A healing process will clean psychological debris as well as physical toxins from the body.

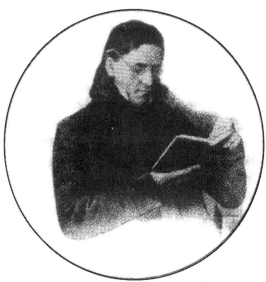

Constantine Hering

To be physically healthy, you must also be mentally and emotionally healthy. Our thoughts, actions, reactions, and interactions with others have a great bearing on our physical health. Anger, fear, greed, hate, and other negative feelings affect the function of body and secretion of hormones. Such feelings cause hypertension, stress, nervousness, and secretion of too much epinephrine (adrenaline) and other hormones. Excess acid is also produced. The production of too much acid in the body may lead to acidosis. Acidosis creates an environment in the body that is susceptible to numerous degenerative disease conditions.

Toxins from poor-quality food and putrefying fecal matter in the colon poison the entire body, including the brain. As a result, the emotions are affected. This spawns discontent, anger, moodiness, and impatience, which leads to social and family problems. These problems, in turn, aggravate emotional disturbances that increase the acidity and toxicity of the body. Toxins aggravate emotions, which in turn increase toxicity. The cycle feeds itself, growing worse and worse. Is it any wonder that the divorce rate has risen so high in the past few decades or that crime is also at an all time high?

Emotional disturbances or symptoms are often labeled with such terms as PMS, hyperactivity, learning disability, etc. Some people say they just can't understand why a person, who at one time was very friendly, has over the years become a grumpy old man, or why a woman develops PMS. Children are labeled as hyperactive or learning disabled. Simply cleaning the bowels of toxic debris has brought about remarkable changes in the attitude in people. A complete cleansing can bring about permanent positive changes.

Emotional disturbances are a threat to good health. The body's innate wisdom knows this and will remove emotional problems during the cleansing process. For those people who have had severe emotional crises in their lives, the thought of reexperiencing them is disturbing. This is the time when people are most apt to break down and resume eating poor-quality foods. Perceptions become distorted, feelings of discouragement arise, common sense is overridden, and priorities are realigned. Going on a food binge is a typical way of trying to cope with these feelings. Good health doesn't seem to matter any more. Once these emotions are removed, good sense returns.

Like physical illness, these thoughts and emotions need to be purged from the mind. This can only be done by faithfully remaining on a clean diet. Eating poor-quality food will drive these emotions back into the subconscious, only to resurface later. Get rid of them once and for all by sticking to your cleansing diet and riding out the discomforts.

Cleansing will bring feelings of well-being, cheerfulness, vitality, and positive mental emotional feelings, but the emotional crisis must be passed before this can happen. The person must reexperience many emotional states for him or her to be completely purged. During this time you may feel anger, envy, or uselessness, become irritable and lose willpower—these are all signs of emotional cleansing.

Spouses and family members must be made aware of these conditions. They need to be especially patient during these times, give encouragement, and be positive and loving to help the person over this trying period. They must not overreact to what may appear to be unjustified criticism, nagging, moodiness, and mental abuse. This is only a temporary phase that will soon pass. Keeping in mind that once this emotional crisis has passed, the person will become more positive, more loving, happier, and much more of a joy to be around than they have been for years, which should be ample motivation to endure the short crisis period. Be aware that you may experience several emotional crises before the body has cleansed completely. On the other hand, since we are all different, you may not encounter any emotional irregularities.

In Reverse Order

Hering's Law also states that healing will occur "in reverse order as the symptoms have appeared in the body." What this means is that during the cleansing process, symptoms of illnesses that you have had in the past will return. They will resurface in the reverse order in which they occurred, all the way back to childhood. If you had an infection a year ago, you will reexperience the symptoms, especially if they were suppressed with antibiotics or other drugs.

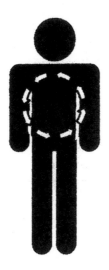

Healing progresses in reverse chronological order, from the most recent illnesses to the oldest.

The idea that past illnesses can return sounds strange to many people. They assume that once an infectious illness is overcome, the microorganism that caused it has been totally vanquished. This is not always so. Pathogenic microorganisms can live hidden deep inside of us, kept under control by our immune system. At times people suffer relapses from diseases that have lain dormant in their cells for many years. Shingles, as an example, is caused by the chicken pox virus. About three percent of the population will suffer from shingles at some time in their lives. In most cases, the disease results from reactivation of the chicken pox virus that lay dormant for years after the original chicken pox infection. It usually resurfaces in older adults after experiencing stress, undergoing radiation therapy, or taking immunosuppressive drugs.

Your fat cells, encrusted mucus, and fecal debris in your intestinal tract represent the chemistry of the body at the time they were formed. Drugs, toxins, harmful microbes, etc. trapped in this material will be released into the bloodstream as the body cleans itself. These substances will cause a reoccurrence of symptoms of disease associated with these toxins.

Because toxic material is emulsified in reverse order in which it formed in the body, the corresponding illnesses will reoccur in reverse order from when they first appeared. The most recent will be the first to resurface. For example, if you had a strep infection eight months ago and a bout with the flu two months ago, you will reexperience the flu first and then the strep infection. Keep in mind that the body has already made antibodies to fight these microbes, so if symptoms appear they will be quickly taken care of by the immune system. In many cases, few or no symptoms will occur. However, if the immune system is weak, as it is with many people, symptoms may be as severe as when the infection first occurred, but will eventually subside without medication. If the body has been cleansing for a while and a healthy lifestyle is being lived, the body will be stronger and better able to repel any resurfacing illnesses.

Typically, when a person who is on a cleansing program reexperiences an illness, the first thought is that he or she "caught" another infection. Often, the treatment is blamed for weakening the body to such a point that sickness occurred. Keep in mind that this infection is not a new one, but a purging of an old one. The person's body is becoming stronger and is throwing off all remnants of the microbe or chemicals (drugs, poisons, toxins) that caused the illness. The infection will be short lived. Suppressing the illness with drugs, however, would drive the bacteria or toxins back into the tissues where they were before. These agents of dis-ease would again need to be brought out through a cleansing crisis. Drugs hamper the body's cleansing processes. If an infection resurfaces, it is best treated with natural, user-friendly medications such as herbs.

As people age, often their immune systems become overworked. Stress, toxic accumulation, and infections may all contribute to weakening of the immune system. As a result, old microbes and toxic debris trapped in the tissues of the body are allowed to reinfect the system. These can cause great harm. Unlike the release of toxins during a cleaning crisis when the body has become strong enough to purge the poisons from the system, a degenerating body is weak and a disease crises arises, causing repeated illness and continual discomfort. The entire body breaks down and deteriorates until disease overcomes it. Healing the body through a cleansing process will help keep this from happening.

In his book *Juicing Therapy,* Bernard Jensen, D.C., Ph.D., relates an experience with a patient who suffered with numerous chronic leg ulcers. She had seen may doctors over the years without success. Dr. Jensen put her on a cleansing diet and detoxification program. Within three weeks her legs were completely healed. She did not go through a healing crisis at this time, but after about three months under his care, this patient lost her sight for two days. At first she could not understand why this should happen, and then she remembered an incident a number of years earlier when, as a piano teacher, she had worked so intensely in preparing for a recital that she lost her sight for two days. After two days, her sight was restored to the state when the disorder began.

Another lady had extreme scoliosis (curvature of the spine). During detoxification she developed what she described as a severe cold. Afterward her spine was remarkably better and continued to improve. Some people will experience severe back pain for several days or even for a couple of weeks, but after that the pain will suddenly disappear, their posture will be improved, they will stand taller, and they will have more flexibility.

If you had back problems in the past, pain may temporarily return as the body heals and adjusts to overcome structural problems.

A person who suffered dizzy spells and headaches ever since being in a car accident as a teenager reported a disappearance of these symptoms after a healing crisis. Symptoms increased briefly during the crisis, but she reported afterward that she has remained symptom-free for months.

If you have had dental problems, your teeth may hurt. You may reencounter stabbing pain extending down to the nerve and feel it is infected. The body is healing; you don't need to have any dental work at this time. Your teeth are removing bacteria, inflammations, etc., and although swelling may occur and it may hurt to chew, it will heal on its own in a few days.

Sore feet, earaches, arthritis, ulcers, ringworm, and any other problem may resurface or intensify temporarily during the crisis as cleansing is taking place. A full recovery may not happen after one crisis, but symptoms may be improved. If the condition has been present for many years, it will take time to completely correct it. Some people may have to experience dozens of healing crises over several years to cleanse and remove a lifetime of toxic accumulation.

CHAPTER 7

HEALING CRISIS VERSUS
DISEASE CRISIS _____ ■

The Differences Between
Healing and Disease Crises

One of the most often asked questions about the healing crisis is how does one distinguish the difference between a healing crisis and a disease crisis? The healing crisis manifests the same type of symptoms as the disease crisis. In both cases the body is removing toxins and cleansing itself, so both are cleansing crises. In a healing crisis, however, the body is becoming stronger and healthier. In a disease crisis, the body is struggling to remove toxic levels of poisons and microbial infestations in an effort just to survive.

A disease crisis develops when toxins accumulating in the body have reached a level of concentration where the immune system cannot adequately handle them and normal body functions, and in some cases life itself, are threatened.

As a result, the body reacts with a heavy cleansing crisis. A crisis is a signal for the body to stop and rest. Typically, symptoms of illness include a discharge from one or more organs of elimination along with aches, pains, a lack of energy, and a loss of appetite. Often, just the thought of certain foods will cause feelings of nausea. The reason the body brings on these symptoms is not only as a means to remove toxins, but to tell the mind it needs to take time to rest and to cut down the intake of foods. The body needs rest so that it can focus its energy on cleansing. Food intake needs to be reduced, not only to prevent more toxins from entering the body, but to conserve energy that would be spent in digestion.

The disease crisis comes on after a gradual buildup of toxins from food, drugs, environmental pollutants, or microorganisms. It can also occur as a result of a weakening of the immune system from physical or emotional stress. How often have you caught a cold during a stressful time in your life: finals at school, heavy workload, or family or social troubles? The disease crisis occurs to save life.

The healing crisis is a product of natural laws. It comes only when you do the things that promote good health. The body was programmed to function in harmony with the laws of nature to maintain optimal health. When you do things to support that goal, your body will work toward this end. If you subject yourself to harmful influences and poor lifestyle choices, health declines, and healing crises do not occur. Therefore, before you can have a healing crisis, you must be actively improving your health.

Let's say someone has been on a natural health program for six months and becomes "sick," how can you tell if it is a disease crises or a healing crisis? If the person has been removing toxins and diseased tissues for six months and replacing them with strong healthy cells, the body is much stronger and healthier than it has been. The channels of elimination have improved. The immune system has improved. The person has more energy. Powers of recuperation are stronger. Remember, a disease crisis occurs when toxic levels build up to a point that the body goes into a state of distress, resulting in massive elimination to prevent further damage. If the person is now stronger, healthier, and has more vital energy than before, the cleansing crisis he encounters is probably a healing crisis.

However, if a person has been on a detoxification program for only a month when he has a crisis, is it a healing crisis or a illness? One month is often not long enough to completely clean and repair the body. A person with years of accumulation of toxins and environmental pollutants cannot clean out this mess in just one month. Channels of elimination will still be more sluggish than normal. The immune system will still be overburdened. So how can you tell?

Illness can't tackle a body that is strong and healthy, or if it does, it will not last long. As you eat right and live right, your body becomes stronger, tissues and cells become stronger, and organs become more efficient. Waste and toxins are removed more efficiently, so a disease crisis should not be manifest except, perhaps, on rare occasions.

A disease crisis may happen, however, if you are exposed to more negative influences than you can handle, whether you are on a cleansing program or not. If you sneak "treats," take medications, use external chemicals on the skin (e.g., antiperspirants, chemical-laden lotions and shampoos, etc.), are in contact with environmental pollutants, undergoing excessive stress, or frequently exposed to contagious microorganisms, the effects are accumulative and illness may result. If the flu is going around, you may catch it because of constant exposure to the flu virus and other negative influences that weaken your immune system. If the flu is not affecting those around you, and you come down with flu-like symptoms while on a cleansing program, it is more than likely a healing crisis.

The body continually works to achieve homeostasis— where every organ functions in harmony with each other to establish a physiological equilibrium. According to Bernard Jensen, Ph.D., a renowned authority in natural health and the healing crisis, for a healing crisis to develop, the organs have to reach a state of integrity where they can accomplish the functions for which they were designed. Every organ has become healthier, and elimination has reached an improved level of efficiency. They may not be completely healthy yet, but they are working better than they had before. When all organs are strong enough to do the job of elimination, toxins will be purged. A healing crisis brings on elimination through all five of the eliminating organs— skin, bowel, lungs, liver, and kidneys. The elimination in a healing crisis is greater than that in a disease crisis because each of these organs are working more efficiently. The colon, for example, in a healing crisis has reached a state of health where it is able to handle the task of elimination. During a disease crisis, the colon is weak and toxins are not efficiently removed, causing fecal matter to become trapped in the bowels where it putrefies and poisons the system. That is why enemas are often recommended for those who are sick. However, you don't necessarily need an enema during a healing crisis because the colon is healthier and more capable of handling the workload.

Before a healing crisis strikes, the body has been healing and getting stronger. You will feel a sense of well-being. Often you will experience a burst of energy and renewed vitality immediately before a crisis strikes. The crisis initiates intense cleansing and rebuilding accompanied with symptoms of elimination and, often, discomfort. After the healing crisis, you will again have a feeling of health and well-being. You may experience several healing crises and feel better and better after each one. Disease crises, on the other hand, can linger on and sap your strength for an extended time even after the worst symptoms have faded. You feel no improvement in health after the crisis than you did before.

Symptoms and Drugs

When a person first encounters a severe healing crisis, it is common to worry. Even though well informed about the discomforts of the healing process, the person doesn't really believe, accept, or understand it. What often happens is that the person begins to wonder if the crisis is really a disease crisis. If it is a disease crisis, the person may feel a need to get medical attention so it doesn't get worse. After all, medical doctors are well trained to handle emergencies and life threatening situations. The discomfort of the crisis may get worse with each day. The person worries and begins to believe that it must be an illness and medical help is needed. The person goes to the doctor. If you go to a doctor what can he do for you? Diagnosing an illness won't cure it. All the doctor will do is give you some drugs to suppress the symptoms.

Symptoms are necessary for the removal of toxins. They are the body's means of healing. During a disease crisis the symptoms are not the disease; they are the reactions of the body to disease. Stopping the symptoms does not cure the disease.

We have been conditioned all our lives to believe that when we get sick, we must go to the doctor for something to make us feel better. We are continually blasted with this theology in advertisements. "For fast pain relief get...." "To soothe aching muscles use...." "For relief of upset stomach buy...." There seems to be a "cure" for just about any ailment, or at least that is the concept we are led to believe by the drug companies. We are conditioned to want and expect instant relief. Natural healing doesn't work that way. It takes time. Drugs that suppress symptoms will give a false sense of being cured as a war rages on deep inside the body.

The body was designed to heal itself. You get a cut, there is nothing you can do to heal it. You might put something on it to keep out infection, or if it is deep, apply a bandage to stop bleeding; but that is about all you can do. The body does the healing. The same is true for any injury or illness. If you catch a cold or get an infection, there is nothing you can do to heal the body. There are medications (both natural and chemical) that you can take that may help, but it is the body's innate wisdom and curative power that eventually brings healing.

The body has to heal itself whether it is encumbered with drugs or not. It can usually do a better job of healing without the added burden of dealing with toxic chemicals. The body does the healing, *not* the doctor and *not* the drugs. Taking medications during a cleansing crisis to treat symptoms stops the cleansing process.

If a viral or bacterial infection results from a healing crisis, it is because the infection is being pulled out of the tissues. This means you have been exposed to it before and your immune system has already made antibodies that will eventually overpower and completely eradicate the infectious agents. Drugs won't help.

Even if you were going through a disease crisis, taking drugs may not help. They will suppress the symptoms without treating the cause. So it doesn't really matter whether you are going through a disease crisis or a healing crisis, taking drugs to mask the symptoms will only make matters worse. If symptoms are severe and you feel that you need something, try natural herbal remedies first. A natural health care practitioner or personnel at your local health food store can show you what products work best. They are harmless when taken at suggested dosages and may do you some good. The time when drugs, such as antibiotics, are useful is during a severe *disease crisis* when the body is infected by a dangerous bacteria (not a virus—antibiotics are useless against them) and is in such poor health it cannot otherwise muster the strength to fight off the infection. This is the type of person who pays little attention to diet or health. Unfortunately, most people have such poor dietary and lifestyle habits that their bodies often need these types of drugs to survive. But practicing preventative medicine by eating healthfully and cleansing out toxins will give the body the strength it needs to fight most infections without resorting to drugs.

The healing crisis must be understood before you try any natural healing or detoxification program. You only get better, not sicker. The healing crisis is a sign of improving health and needs no help from medications or other treatments. The reason the crisis has arisen is because the body has become strong enough to throw off the toxins and remove them from the tissues, and elimination organs have become strong enough to handle the removal. Look forward to the healing crisis and rejoice when it happens. Although you may feel bad physically and perhaps mentally for a while, you will know that you are healing and will have improved health when it is over.

The Garbage Can Model of Disease

Throughout life our bodies collect and store toxins. These toxins slowly poison our bodies, leading to degeneration and poor health. Our level of health depends on how much toxic debris we hold. Symptoms associated with toxic buildup include frequent sickness (i.e., cold, flu, pneumonia), fatigue, insomnia, aches and pains, headaches, constipation, depression, skin blemishes (i.e., psoriasis, rashes, liver spots), bad breath, body odor, digestive problems, mental deterioration, etc. Degenerative diseases like cancer, heart disease, and diabetes are also influenced by the level of toxins in our bodies.

Why are some people sick all the time while others rarely are? Why do some people suffer with cancer, arthritis, and other degenerative diseases while others don't? How can some people with chronic health problems or life threatening diseases reclaim their health even after conventional medicine has failed?

I like to explain this through what I call "The Garbage Can Model of Disease." This analogy explains in a graphic way why we get sick. It also describes the relationship between toxic load, the healing crisis, and the disease crisis.

In this analogy the body can be viewed as a container, like a garbage can, that collects and holds sewage and waste. This garbage represents all the toxic substances that enter and accumulate in our bodies during our lifetime (Figure 1).

Throughout life our bodies (our garbage cans) are filled with sewage and waste. This garbage comes from harmful substances in the food we eat, the liquids we drink, the air we breathe, things in our environment that are absorbed

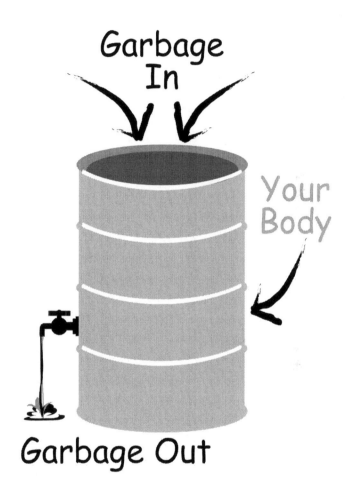

Figure 1

through our skin, and processes inside our bodies. As this toxic waste builds up, our health gets worse and worse. When the container is filled to the top, it has reached its maximum capacity. It can't hold any more and overflows. This is the equivalent of death. The faster our garbage can fills, the sooner we die.

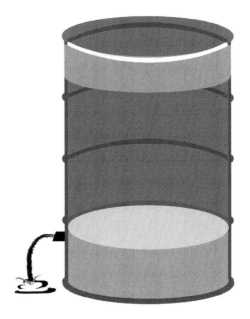

Figure 2

Since we are constantly bombarded with toxins from our environment and the production of metabolic and cellular waste within us, life would be very short unless there was some way to remove these toxins. Fortunately, there is. A release valve located near the bottom of our container provides a way to expel garbage as it accumulates (Figure 2). The release valve represents our body's natural processes of elimination. Our body works constantly to remove or drain the toxins we accumulate every day. Toxins are neutralized and expelled though the bowels, kidneys, liver, skin, etc.

As long as we aren't exposed to more toxins than our bodies can expel, we do okay. If toxins accumulate too fast, they can fill the container quickly, resulting in disease and a short lifespan. However, our trashcans are equipped with a series of release valves (Figure 3). If garbage begins to fill up faster than the main (lowest) release valve can remove it, the pressure triggers the next highest release valve to open to quickly expel as much garbage as possible and avoid overflowing. We call this event a *sickness* or a

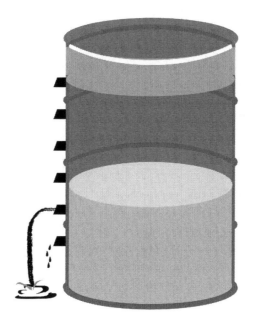

Figure 3

disease crisis. During this time we feel terrible. We may experience diarrhea, nausea, vomiting, sinus discharge, bad breath, fever and sweating, and so forth, all processes in which the body neutralizes and eliminates toxins.

In a disease crisis the body is thrown into a state of panic because it is threatened by death if it doesn't quickly release accumulated toxins. The immune system is thrust into a heightened level of activity, represented by the second release valve opening. When the garbage level in the container drops below the release valve, the discharge and cleansing symptoms stop.

We have many release valves going up the side of our garbage can. If a lower release valve does not open, garbage continues to build and climbs higher and higher inside the can. Eventually it reaches a point at which another release valve, higher up on the side of the can, kicks open and the toxins evacuate. In time, this release valve may also become clogged and refuse to open. In that case, the garbage is forced to pile up even higher. Over time, garbage accumulates to higher and higher levels, slowly creeping towards the brim.

What causes release valves to clog? There are many causes. Some of which include:

- Poor diet (lack of good nutrition)
- Excessive stress
- Inadequate fluid intake (dehydration)
- Lack of exercise
- Lack of adequate sunshine
- Drugs
- Age

Yes, even age affects these release valves. Like it or not, as we age, our bodies just don't function as effectively as they used to. So age will eventually reduce the effectiveness of the

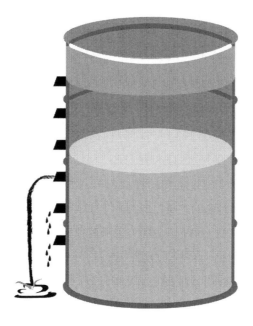

Figure 4

release valves. Most of the other factors are associated with lifestyle choices.

As the release valves become less and less efficient, garbage slowly accumulates higher and higher. Even when a release valve is forced to open during a sickness, toxic waste isn't drained completely. The result is that the sewage in the garbage can remains at an elevated level (Figure 4).

When toxins in the container build up, you begin to experience more illness and develop chronic health problems. The toxic load in your garbage can begins to rot your container (body). The result is the development of degenerative disease like arthritis, osteoporosis, dementia, and so forth. As release valves continue to become clogged and garbage mounts, health begins to deteriorate until the container overflows and we die (Figure 5).

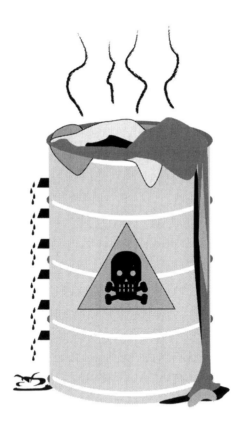

Figure 5

When our trash cans hold a small load of garbage, we are healthy. This usually occurs in our youth. As the garbage can begins to fill, our health declines. So the level of garbage in our trash cans determines our level of health and the way we feel (Figure 6).

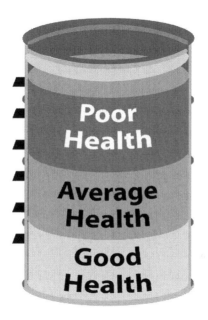

Figure 6

Occasionally we are exposed to large amounts of harmful substances in a short amount of time. This occurs when we come into contact with massive dose of poison, such as lead, or disease-causing bacteria. If our garbage can is nearly full, the addition of the contaminant may be enough to quickly fill the can to overflowing, resulting in a life-threatening illness.

If, however, our garbage can is relatively empty, these toxins will temporarily add a heavy load to the can, but the numerous working release valves will quickly expel them. The response will be a period of illness (elimination of the toxins) and then things will get better. If the garbage is very low, the response will be very quick or perhaps there will be few noticeable symptoms at all. This is why during flu season some people get sick and others don't.

The rate at which our garbage cans fill and release waste is to a great extent under our control. There are three things you can do to reduce the amount of garbage in your trash can.

1. Limit exposure to toxins. Reduce the amount of garbage thrown into the trash. Eat foods without chemical additives, drink pure water without chlorine and fluoride, etc.

2. Live a healthy lifestyle. Do those things that keep your release valves in good working order and avoid activities that harm your health. Eat a nutritious diet, exercise regularly, breathe fresh air, get adequate sunshine, etc.

3. Empty the trash! Actively participate in periodic detoxifications.

When you do a detox, you are taking the highest clogged release valve and opening it up, allowing garbage to exit. You, in effect, are removing an entire layer of garbage (Figure 7). What do you suppose happens when a release valve opens and the body rapidly expels toxins? You feel terrible! It's just like a sickness. You may have diarrhea, vomiting, skin outbreaks, sinus congestion, fever, and so on.

This is a healing or cleansing crisis. The symptoms are virtually identical to that of a sickness or disease crisis. However a disease crisis and a healing crisis are opposites.

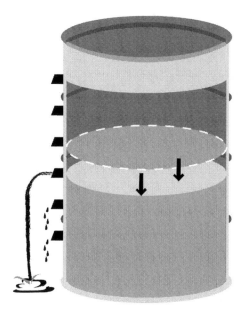

Figure 7

During a sickness your body is struggling to maintain health. During a healing crisis your body is purging toxins to achieve better health. There is a big difference.

After a sickness your body is relieved; it is saved from immediate danger, but you are still no healthier than you were before the sickness. There is no overall improvement.

However, after a healing crisis, your body is rejuvenated. You have just removed an entire layer of poison. Your level of health is now improved. Your toxic level is reduced back to where it was some time ago. It's almost as if time was turned back and you are physically at stage that you were months or years earlier, when you were younger and healthier.

After toxins are released, your garbage level is reduced to a more manageable level. Your risk of developing chronic health problems decreases and health improves. Health problems that may have been present before may now disappear. Please note that you can not remove all the toxins in your body by doing a single detox. Detoxification is a continual process and should be done frequently. As you detox, you unclog and open the highest clogged release valve. The next detox opens the next clogged release valve and so on down the container. As each release valve is opened, a layer of garbage is removed and health improves.

Every time you do a detox that is effective enough to accomplish any good, it will result in a healing crisis. The crisis may be very dramatic and uncomfortable or it may be so mild that you hardly notice any symptoms.

Some people don't like the discomfort associated with detoxification. So they claim it isn't necessary and that a person can heal without it. These people don't understand the healing process and the significance of the healing crisis. They say you can take a slower approach and heal just as well. This, however, is not true. Simply improving your diet may not be enough to bring about changes that would have any significant impact on your health. This is especially true if you have a serious degenerative condition. Simply improving your diet and avoiding harmful influences is good and helpful, but it may not be enough to open that release valve. In this case, improvement can be very, very slow. It may take ten years to achieve the same level of cleansing and improvement that one single healing crisis can bring. You can enjoy ten years of improved health and increased vitality rather than take a slower (less involved) approach. Yes, healing crises are uncomfortable, but if they can give you years of improved health, isn't it worth it?

You don't get any younger as you age. Your release valves become corroded with time, making it harder to expel toxins. If you take the slow approach, you may even die of old age before you see improvement.

A healing crisis or detoxification can be accomplished in many ways. Some methods work faster and better than others. There are several natural methods of detoxification that are designed specifically to cleanse the body of accumulated toxins and bring about better health.* For instance, certain vitamins, minerals, and herbs can stimulate rapid detoxification, allowing the body to flush out huge amounts of toxic debris.

Your Immune System
Keeps You Alive and Healthy

Your immune system and your channels of elimination, the release valves in my analogy, are what keep your body clean and free from disease. When the immune system is working well, we maintain good health. When it is overburdened with toxins, disease and illness result.

When people get sick they often say they "caught" a cold and blame it on a chance encounter with the cold virus. However, germs don't cause sickness. They may be involved, but they don't *cause* it. Coming in contact with a virus or bacteria does not cause illness. Think about it for a moment. Cold and flu viruses are everywhere in our environment. We come into contact with them every single day. If the cold virus caused a cold, everybody on earth would have a cold—all the time. So why doesn't everybody have colds all the time? And why do some people get a cold or the flu while others don't?

---

*For a complete look at how to detox your body using the most effective natural methods, I highly recommend *The Detox Book* by Bruce Fife, N.D. See page 102 for more information.

Germs don't cause illness any more than flies cause garbage. Flies are attracted to garbage, they don't cause it. Likewise, a person full of garbage attracts germs. Cold and flu germs can only grow in a body that is full of garbage. This is because the immune system is so overworked it has difficulty fighting off infections.

Germs that surround us every day are only able to take hold inside of us when our immune systems become overworked. As germs begin to grow, the toxic level inside us reaches a critical point: our bodies go into a state of panic and toxins are flushed as quickly as possible to prevent death. This is a disease crisis.

Chronic illnesses and degenerative diseases are also disease crises. They too, occur as a result of a weakened immune system. We all have degenerative cells in our bodies. Cells wear out, become damaged, get old, and die. Some cells become cancerous. Our immune system cleans these diseased and cancerous cells from our body. Degenerative and cancerous cells are developing constantly, so our immune system must constantly clean them out. If the immune system is overworked it cannot effectively do this job. Diseased or cancerous cells begin to accumulate. The result is degenerative disease and cancer.

From this explanation you can see that a healing crisis is a process in which the body is becoming stronger and healthier. In contrast, a disease crisis is a process in which the body is struggling to survive.

> The physician of tomorrow will be the nutritionist of today.
>
> —Thomas Edison

CHAPTER 8

WHAT TO EXPECT
AND WHAT TO DO _____ ■

What to Expect

Nature's way of purging harmful toxins from the body and restoring health is by way of the healing crisis. Crises can be so mild they are unnoticeable or so dramatic you almost think your life is about to end. In order to remove dis-ease from the body and achieve health and well-being, you must go through the cleansing crisis. Prepare yourself mentally for it. Look forward to it. When it comes, be happy that you are healing.

No two people are alike. Everyone eats differently, has unique genetic makeup, and follows varying lifestyles. Everyone has different levels of health. The symptoms you encounter, their frequency and their severity, will be completely different from those of anyone else. So you can't compare yourself with others.

Often, chronic conditions from which you are suffering will temporarily get worse. If you suffer from arthritis, joint pain may increase. If you are troubled with chronic migraines, you may have terrible headaches. A psoriasis problem may run wild. Hemorrhoids may flair up.

PMS may intensify. Allergies may get worse. Asthmatics may experience breathing difficulties. Blood pressure may increase. Any number of other symptoms could surface during this time that may appear unrelated to existing health conditions. Sometimes these conditions improve after the crisis. Sometimes it takes several crises to cleanse the offending toxins from the body and stimulate healing. At times, health problems can improve immediately after a crisis, and at other times, they improve gradually.

The crisis can come without warning, but generally you will know it is close at hand by the way you feel. You will have a surge of energy and a greater sense of well-being just before the crisis. This is how it usually works. The eliminatory organs become stronger and more efficient, energy level increases and you feel great, better than you have for months. Cleansing and rebuilding are proceeding at an accelerated pace. This explosion of activity can only come about when the body is strong enough to handle intensive housecleaning. Then the bottom drops out. The body pulls out so much junk that has been stored in the tissues that unpleasant symptoms appear.

The first healing crisis will come according to the health of the individual. A young person may have a crisis after only a couple of weeks, while for an elderly person it may take three months or more. Older people have the effects of many more years of poor living habits to correct than younger ones. So, generally, the older you are, the more severe and more frequent crises will be.

The type of healing program you use will also determine the speed of healing and cleansing. Fasting, for example, is one of the quickest methods of cleansing and can easily initiate a healing crisis.

A healing crisis can come as a result of anything you do that improves your health and strengthens the immune system. Converting to a natural foods diet and eliminating your exposure to low-quality foods and environmental toxins can bring on a healing crisis. Subclinically malnourished people who take vitamin and mineral supplements have overcome their deficiencies and gone through crises. One supplement dealer commented that he encountered many people who would use his products for a few weeks, then stop because they claimed that they made them sick. The supplements didn't make them sick, they made them healthy enough to purge disease-causing toxins from their bodies. They made themselves sick from their lifestyle and dietary habits. They did not recognize the cleansing crisis for what it was and interpreted it as a sickness.

What to Do

Some people, when they experience their first healing crisis, think it's a disease crisis and give up saying, "The diet didn't work—I got sicker." You can't expect to clean 40 years of junk and rebuild an entire body in just a few weeks. Some health care workers estimate that it takes seven years to thoroughly clean toxins out of the body and rebuild with new healthy tissues. During this time, periodic healing crises should be expected. To some people, seven years may seem like a long time, but as the body cleanses and rebuilds, strength and vitality will continue to increase. Within months you can experience a remarkable improvement in health. Annoying symptoms depart, but complete healing takes time. While detoxing, you do not grow older and sicker, but functionally younger and healthier. You may see improvements in your health almost immediately. The longer you eat wisely and utilize detoxification methods, the healthier you will be. If you return to habits that burden the body with poisons and pollution, good health cannot be maintained.

One of the biggest misconceptions people face with the healing crisis is the belief that they have caught some hideous infection. If they go to a doctor who is not familiar with this aspect of natural healing, he will diagnose it as an allergy or infection and will prescribe antibiotics or other drugs that suppress the healing process. Although the drugs may bring temporary relief, the cleansing process will be halted, and toxins will remain in the body and be reabsorbed into the tissue. To eliminate these toxins, the person must go through the cleansing crisis all over again.

The symptoms of cleansing are part of a curing process and are constructive. Don't try to stop them with medications. Vitamins and natural herbal supplements, however, may be beneficial and can even speed healing, but they are not necessary. Let nature take its course. If you are eating properly, these symptoms are not deficiency conditions or allergic reactions. The symptoms generally will last only a few days to a week or so. If possible, during this time, no drugs should be taken, as the body is trying to eliminate toxins. Taking drugs will only hamper the elimination process and just add more toxins into your system.

So what do you do when a crisis strikes? You don't need to do anything special other than slow down and allow the body to cleanse and heal. Listen to your body. One wise person described his experience and how he reacted: "I developed a nagging headache, pain in my neck and back, lack of energy, dry mouth, and depressed appetite. The symptoms began Sunday afternoon and gradually intensified, reaching a climax on Tuesday. Knowing that symptoms are the body's way of communicating and healing, I tried to follow what my body was telling me.

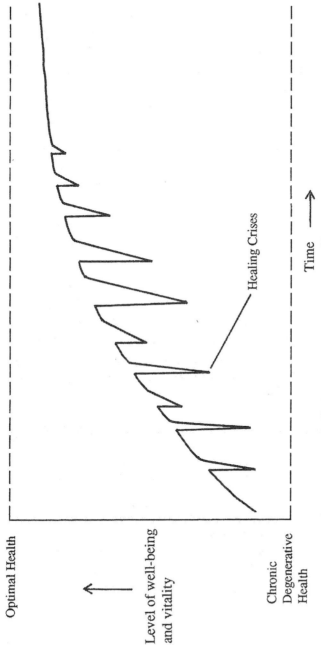

Graphic illustration showing the gradual improvement of health separated by periods of intense cleansing. The degree and duration of cleansing varies with each crisis. Total adherence to a healthful lifestyle, eating wholesome foods, and the advoidance and removal of toxins will produce a health curve similar to that represented above. Negative influences on health pulls the curve down toward chronic degeneration.

Normally I exercise every morning, but because I felt unusually fatigued, I refrained from exercise for a couple of days, and I slept a little longer than normal. Since my mouth was dry, my body was telling me I needed to increase my fluid intake to wash away toxins, so I drank more than usual. And I ate less. I relaxed in a tub of hot water to ease tension in my back. By Tuesday night I started to feel better. Wednesday morning all the symptoms had gone. I felt my normal self, not particularly better or worse than I had before the cleansing crisis. But when I went to exercise that morning, I did notice one new development. My eyesight was dramatically improved. I still needed glasses to get around, but I was able to see things in clear detail that were fuzzy shapes just days before."

The symptoms you develop during a crisis will guide you as to what to do. If you are tired—rest. If you are thirsty—drink. If you have a fever, your body is trying to build up heat, so keep yourself warm and let the heat run its course. For aching muscles, a warm bath might help. Pain in the lower back is often caused by the kidneys

---

Nutritional and biological modalities—diets, vitamins, juices, herbs, etc...are not offered as cures for disease, but only as supportive means of helping the body's own inherent healing forces and assisting its own healing activity. I wish to stress the fact that no food, no vitamin, no herb—and, for that matter, no drug!—can ever cure disease. Disease can be cured only by the body's own healing and health-restoring power.

—Paavo Airola, Ph.D.

crying out for water rather than being the result of sore back muscles. Drink more water. If you have diarrhea or are vomiting, the body is trying to empty itself, so don't try to eat. You will lose fluids, so you should try to drink water to keep from becoming dehydrated. Drinking lots of water during a crisis is usually a good practice because water will help to dilute the toxins in the bloodstream and aid their removal. Mucus becomes more runny when you are properly hydrated. Mucus that becomes thick when you are dehydrated is harder to eliminate and can plug the pipes draining sewage from the body.

Some people notice an increase in body odor and bad breath. The tongue may be coated. These are signs of cleansing. The tongue shows what is happening with the mucous membranes within the body. If it is coated with a white or grayish film, it signifies the expulsion of toxins taking place throughout the body. This coating and the body odor will go away as the crisis comes to an end. Frequent baths may be advisable during the crisis.

Avoid overeating during this time. Eating does not give you strength. It takes energy from the body to digest food and eliminate waste. Conserve this energy by eating lightly, if at all. If you have no hunger, do not eat. It would be good even to fast, consuming only juice, herbal tea, or vegetable broth. Very little energy is needed to digest these liquids, and the nutrients they contain are easily absorbed.

Definitely avoid exposure to any toxic substances, particularly in foods. Avoid processed foods and sweets and convenience foods with food additives (such as preservatives, dyes, flavor enhancers, and other chemicals). Avoid as much as possible polluted air. Sugar depresses the immune system, which is the powerhouse behind the healing crisis. Eating sugary foods and drinks (including too much sweet fruit juice) will weaken the immune response and slow down or even stop the cleansing. Herbs can give the body a boost and aid in the cleansing or help to ease discomfort without hampering the cleansing that is taking place. For advice on the proper use of herbs, talk to a health care worker knowledgeable in this subject. Let the process run its course without interference.

By listening to your body and following its cues, the cleansing action will proceed more quickly and with less trauma. Think positively. Be happy. You are on the threshold of achieving a higher level of health and vitality.

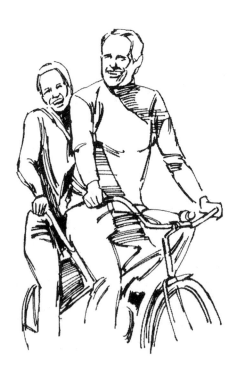

INDEX

THE DETOX BOOK
How to Detoxify Your Body to Improve Your Health, Stop Disease and Reverse Aging

by Bruce Fife, ND

We live in a toxic world. Environmental pollution and disease causing germs assault us continually day after day. Our food is nutrient deficient and our water supply dangerously contaminated. People today are exposed to chemicals in far greater concentrations than were previous generations. Thousands of tons of man-made chemicals and industrial pollutants are poured into our environment and our food supply daily.

With such a massive attack on our health we should all be sick from toxic overload. And we are! In no other time in the history of the world has degenerative disease been as prominent as it is today. Diseases that were rare or unheard of a century ago are now raging upon us like a plague. Millions are dying from diseases that were virtually unknown in the past.

Nature, however, has provided us with the solution. Our bodies are amazingly resilient. If the disease-causing toxins are removed, the body will heal itself. This book outlines the steps you need to take to thoroughly detoxify and cleanse your body from these disease-causing agents. You will also learn how to reduce your toxic exposure and how to strengthen your immune system.

Through detoxification you will free yourself from the chains of pain, reverse degenerative conditions, gain more energy, feel and look younger, improve your memory, and be happier. Virtually all the diseases of modem society, including many infectious illnesses, can be avoided or even cured by sensible systematic detoxification.

Although we live in a toxic world we can take control of our health. This book will show you how.

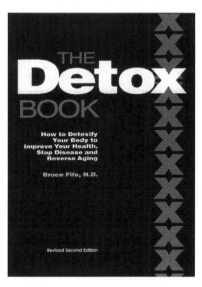

"The Detox Book is highly recommended for health reference collections."

- The Midwest Book Review

" A comprehensive handbook of detoxification therapies... Chapters give extensive background information on each subject, report of research, and precise, detailed instructions for self-administration...An encyclopedic look at how we can care for and cleanse our amazingly resilient bodies."

- Booklist, American Library *Association*

Free Catalog and Newsletter

For more information about **The Detox Book** and other books and materials by Bruce Fife, N.D. write and ask for a free copy of the *Healthy Ways Catalog*. If you would like to learn more about the healing crisis, nutrition, and natural health write or call and ask for a free copy of the *Healthy Ways Newsletter*. Send your request to Piccadilly Books, P.O. Box 25203, Colorado Springs, CO 80936, or call (719)550-9887.

COCONUT WATER FOR HEALTH AND HEALING

Coconut water is a refreshing beverage that comes from coconuts. It's a powerhouse of nutrition containing a complex blend of vitamins, minerals, amino acids, carbohydrates, antioxidants, enzymes, health enhancing growth hormones, and other phytonutrients.

Because its electrolyte (ionic mineral) content is similar to human plasma, it has gained international acclaim as a natural sports drink for oral rehydration. As such, it has proven superior to commercial sports drinks. Unlike other beverages, it is completely compatible with the human body, in so much that it can be infused directly into the bloodstream. In fact, doctors have used coconut water successfully as an intravenous fluid for over 60 years.

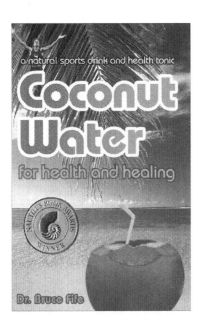

Because of coconut water's unique compatibility with the human body and its nutrient profile, it has proven to be superior to other fruit and vegetable juices in fasting therapy and detoxification.

Coconut water's unique nutritional profile gives it the power to balance body chemistry, ward off disease, fight cancer, and retard aging. History and folklore credit coconut water with remarkable healing powers, which medical science is now confirming. Published medical research and clinical observation have shown that coconut water:

- Makes an excellent oral rehydration sports beverage
- Aids in exercise performance
- Aids in kidney function and dissolves kidney stones
- Protects against cancer
- Provides a source of ionic trace minerals
- Improves digestion
- Contains nutrients that feed friendly gut bacteria
- Helps relieve constipation
- Reduces risk of heart disease
- Improves blood circulation
- Lowers high blood pressure
- Improves blood cholesterol levels
- Helps prevent atherosclerosis
- Prevents abnormal blood clotting
- Possesses anti-aging properties
- Restores strength and elasticity to skin
- Reduces discolored aging spots on skin
- Reduces wrinkles and sagging skin
- Enhances healing of wounds and lesions
- Supports good vision and prevents glaucoma
- Contains potent antioxidants
- Enhances immune function

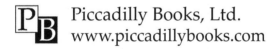 Piccadilly Books, Ltd.
www.piccadillybooks.com

OIL PULLING THERAPY
Detoxifiying and Healing the Body
Through Oral Cleansing

If you have bad breath, bleeding gums, cavities, or tooth pain—you need this book! If you suffer from asthma, diabetes, arthritis, migraine headaches, or any chronic illness, and have not found relief, this book could have the solution for you.

All disease starts in the mouth! As incredible as it may sound, most of the chronic and infectious illnesses that trouble our society today are influenced by the health of our mouths.

Our mouths are a reflection of the health inside our bodies. If you have poor dental health, you are bound to have other health problems. Despite regular brushing and flossing, 98 percent of the population has some degree of gum disease or tooth decay. Most people aren't even aware they have existing dental problems.

All Disease Starts in the Mouth

Oil Pulling Therapy

Detoxifying and Healing the Body Through Oral Cleansing

Dr. Bruce Fife

Recent research has demonstrated a direct link between oral health and chronic illness. Simply improving the health of your teeth and gums can cure many chronic problems.

More brushing, flossing, and mouthwash won't do it. What *will* work is Oil Pulling Therapy. Oil pulling is an age-old method of oral cleansing originating from Ayurvedic medicine. It is one of the most powerful, most effective methods of detoxification and healing in natural medicine.

Dr. Fife's Oil Pulling Therapy is a revolutionary new treatment combining the wisdom of Ayurvedic medicine with modern science. The science behind oil pulling is fully documented with references to medical studies and case histories. Although incredibly powerful, Oil Pulling Therapy is completely safe and simple enough for even a child.

Oil Pulling Therapy guarantees to give you fresher breath, healthier gums, whiter teeth and help protect you from many chronic health problems.

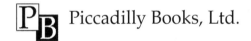 Piccadilly Books, Ltd.